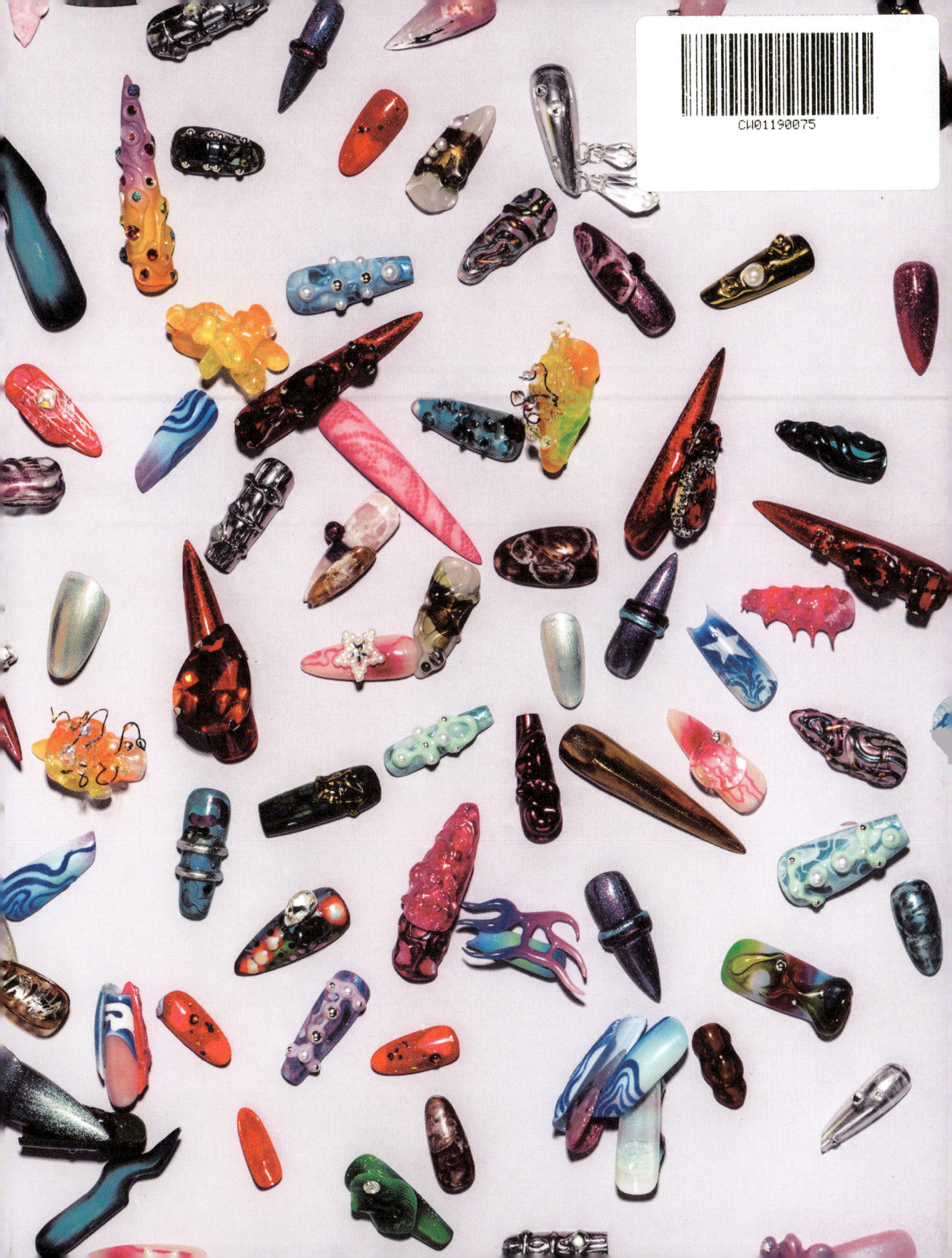

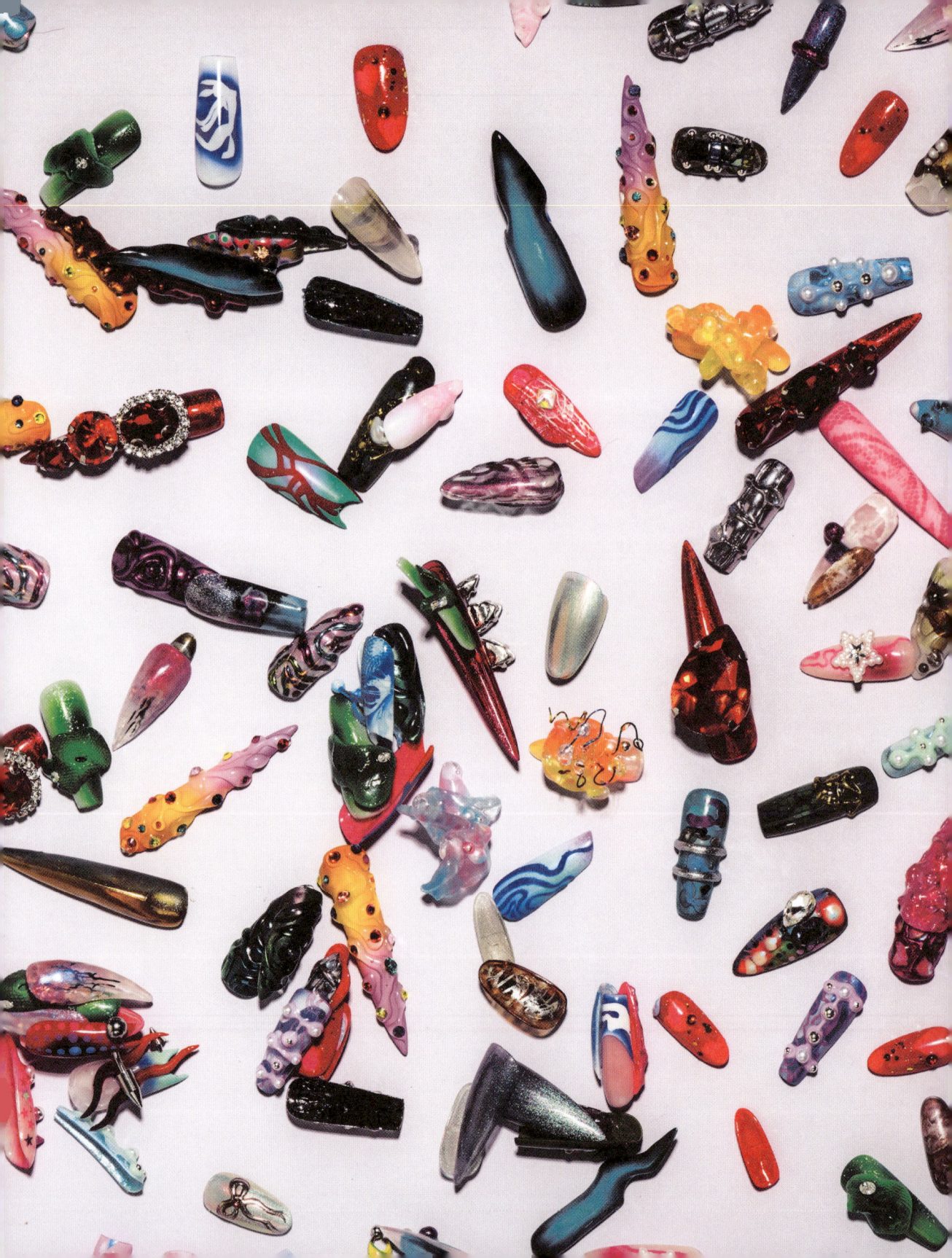

MANNEQUIN HANDS

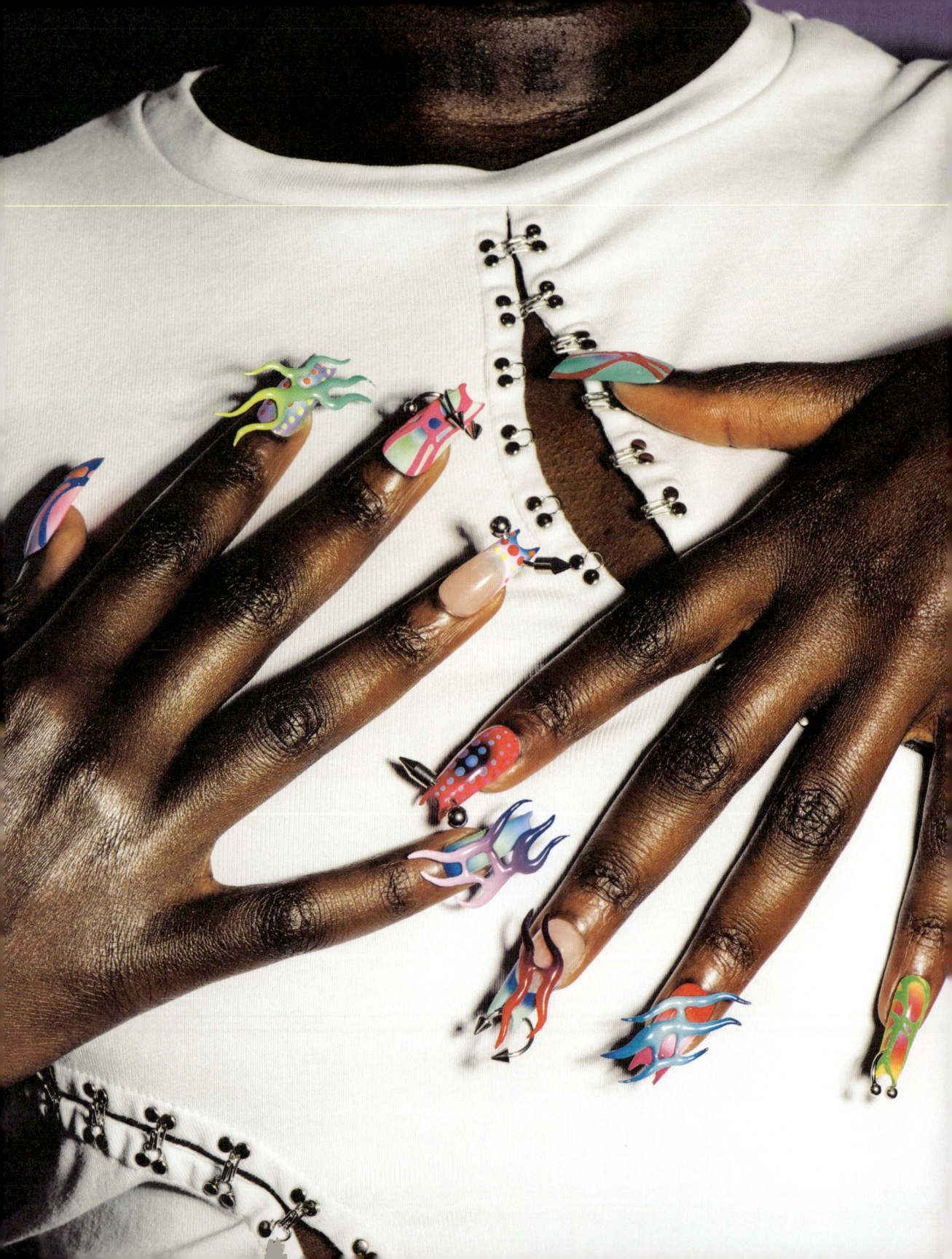

A GUIDE TO NAIL ART

MANNEQUIN HANDS

BY VICTORIA HOULLIS

Sweet Hearts
PRESS

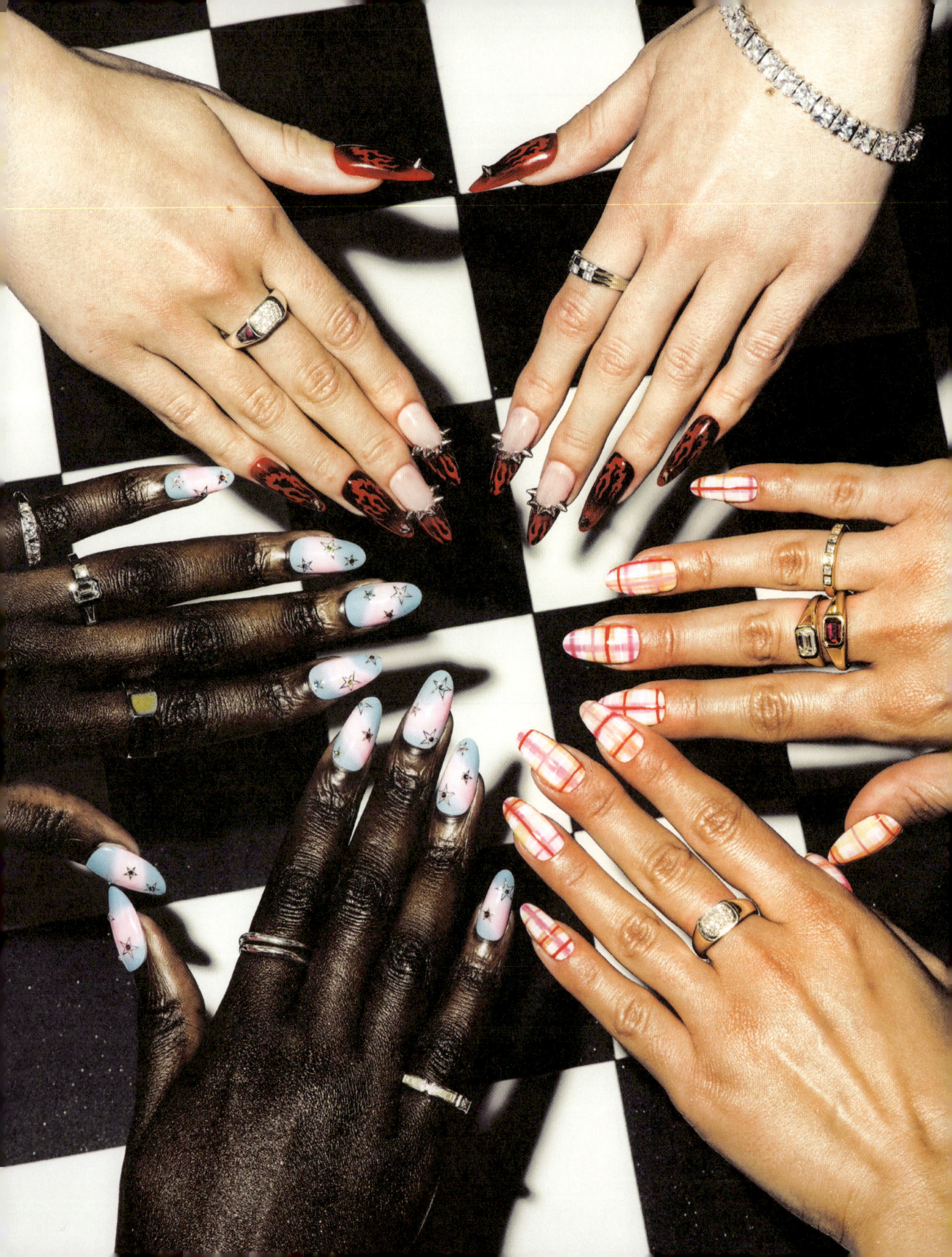

Dedicated to my parents and anyone I've ever had the pleasure of holding hands with.

With gratitude and thanks to the POC who pioneered and championed the beauty of nail art.

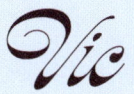

CONTENTS
Contents
CONTENTS
Contents
CONTENTS
Contents

INTRODUCTION	01
NAIL ART NOW	05
MANNEQUIN HANDS SETS	17
THE BASICS	79
HANDS-ON TUTORIALS	107
STICK IT	157
CREATE IT	167
ABOUT THE AUTHOR	192
ACKNOWLEDGEMENTS	196

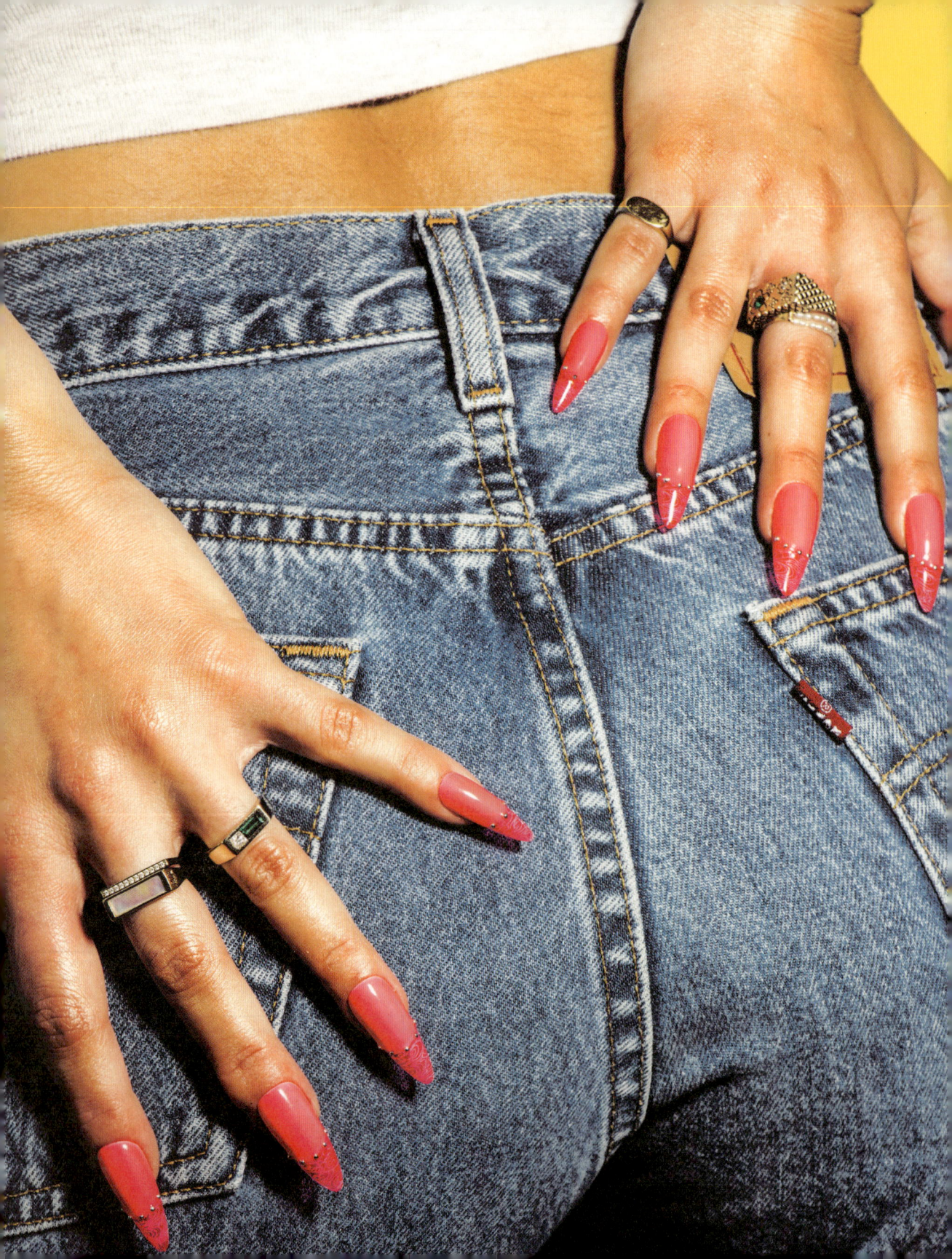

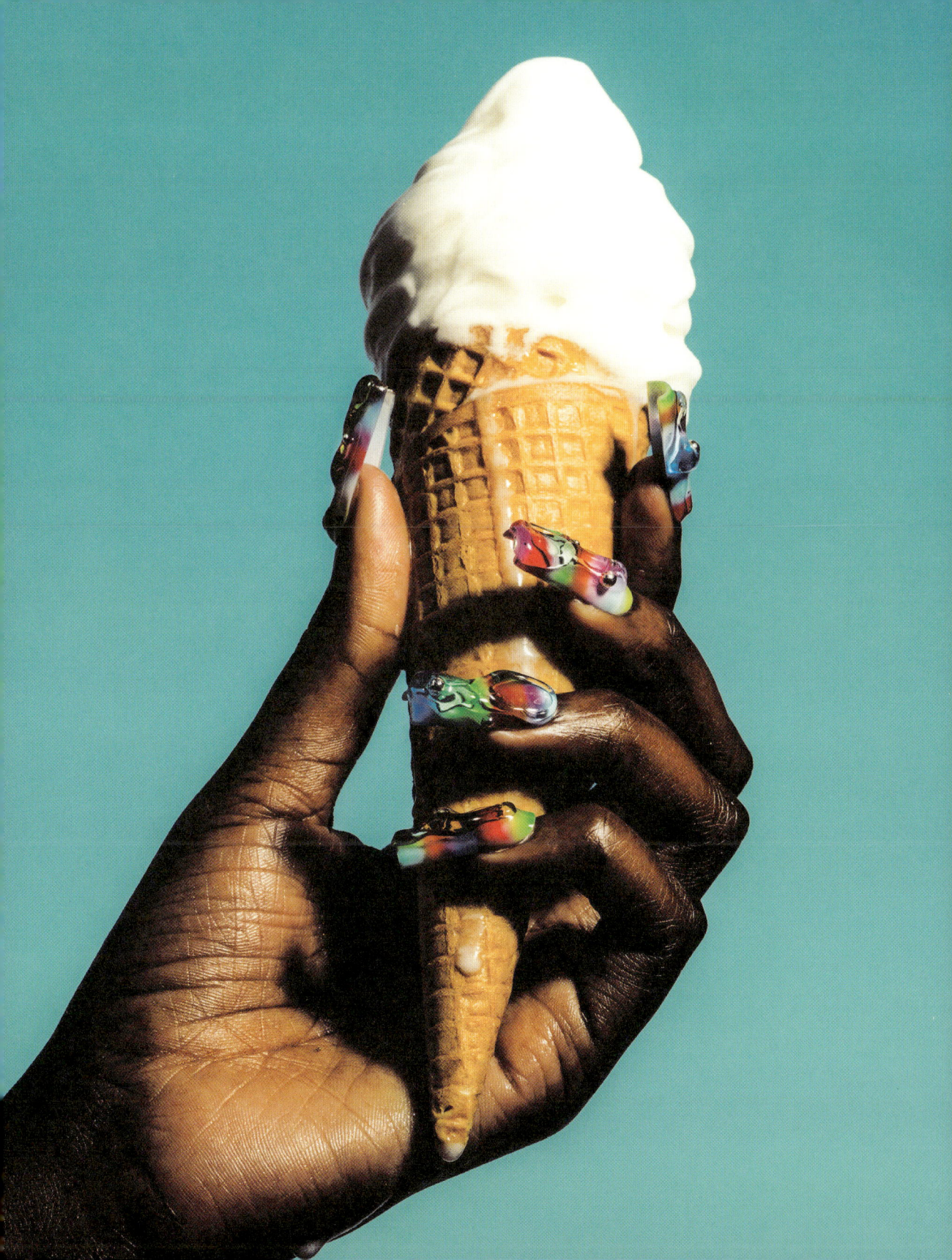

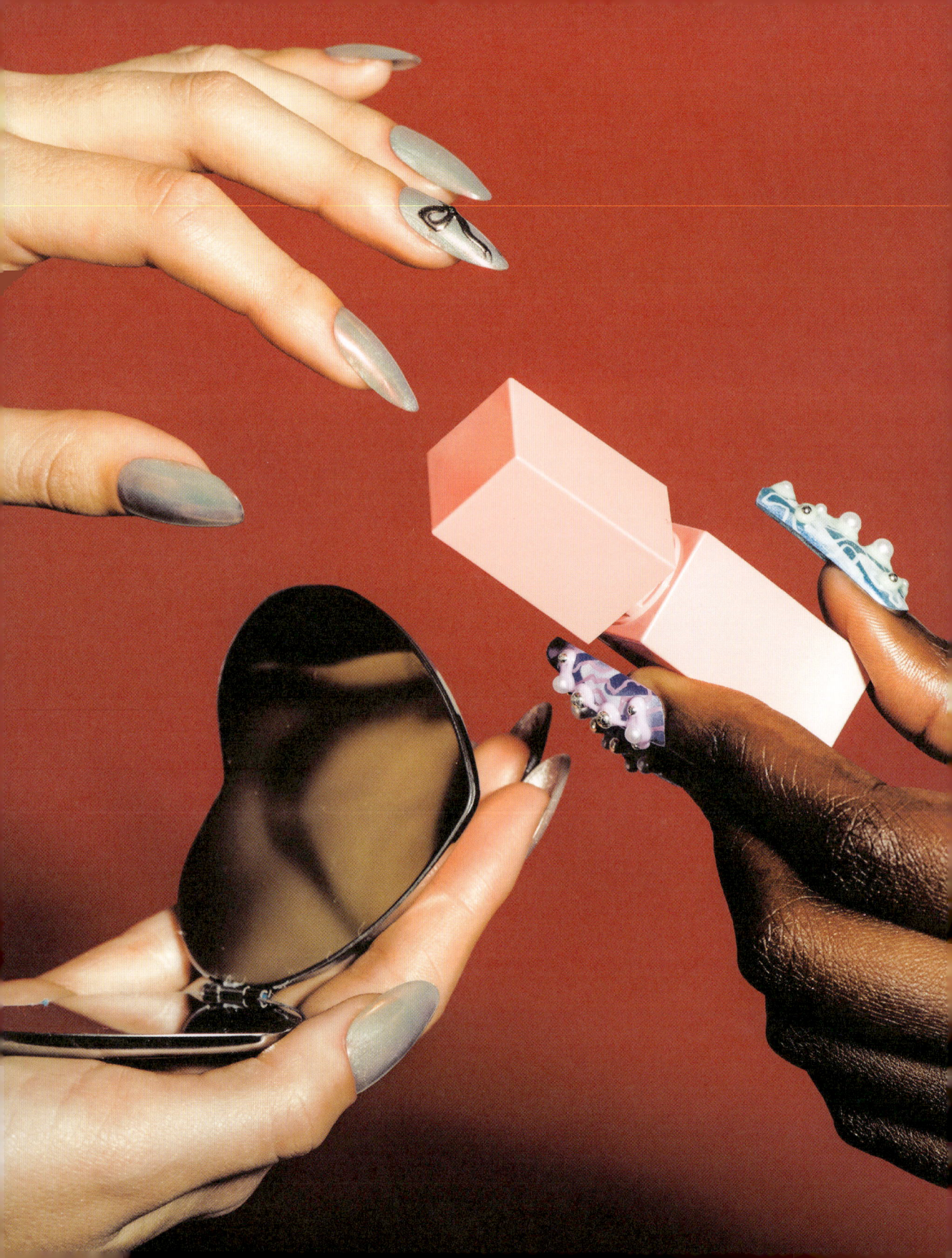

INTRODUCTION

Welcome to my personal guide to nail art. While one book can't quite sum up all the science, technology, skill, passion, creativity, politics and community that make up the world of nail art, this captures some of my thoughts and experiences to help others begin their own journey. The world of nail art is vast, ever-changing and takes up a solid corner of the internet. This book was made to inspire, inform and ignite your love of nail art every time you reach for it. *Mannequin Hands* is my love letter to nail art.

This book is a mix of the technical need-to-know stuff, with some of the biology of nails, the science behind some of the most commonly used nail products and a step-by-step guide that'll teach you how to perform a manicure in the comfort of your own home. If you'd never part hands with your nail tech then this book will give you a solid breakdown of techniques, insights into why your nail tech does 'this or that', how to ask for exactly what you'd like and the best ways to get the most out of your nails.

The book features a collection of curated sets crafted especially to take you on a journey of some of my favourite nail art looks. If you feel like getting hands on with the tools, there's guides on nail art looks that can be achieved at home, along with the processes and products for bringing them to life on your own hands.

There are even stencils at the back of the book where you can map out your future sets. Grab your pencils, pens, markers or paint to conjure up the nail sets of your dreams. For those who love a nail decal, I've crafted a special decal set featuring some of my signature shapes and designs as well as versatile 'must have's' that immediately make the simplest manicure pop!

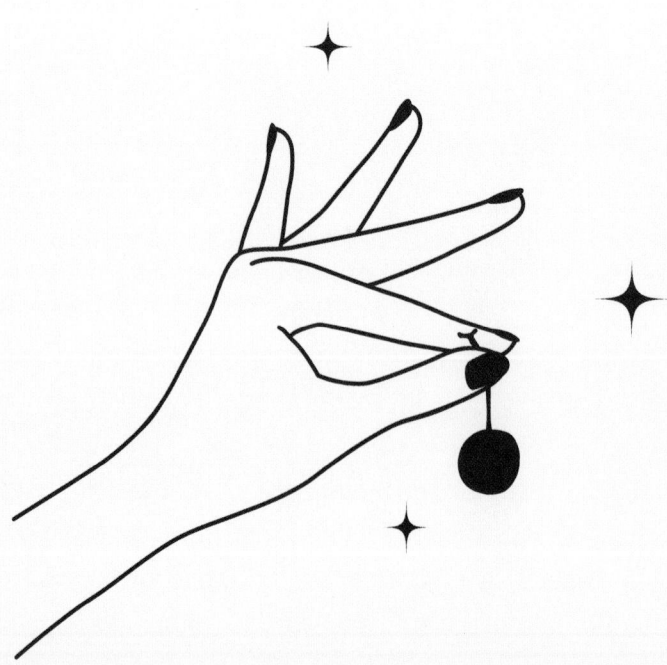

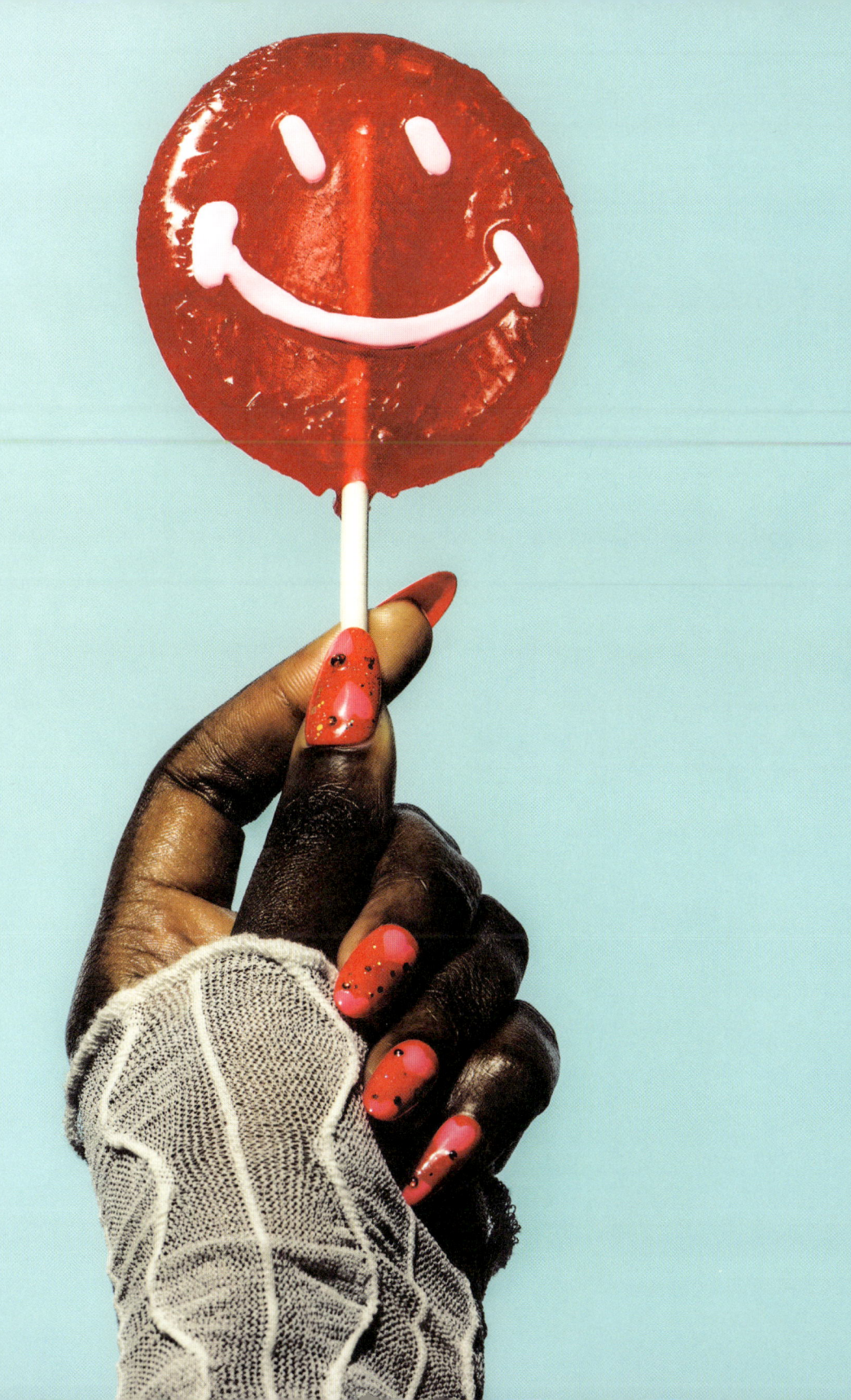

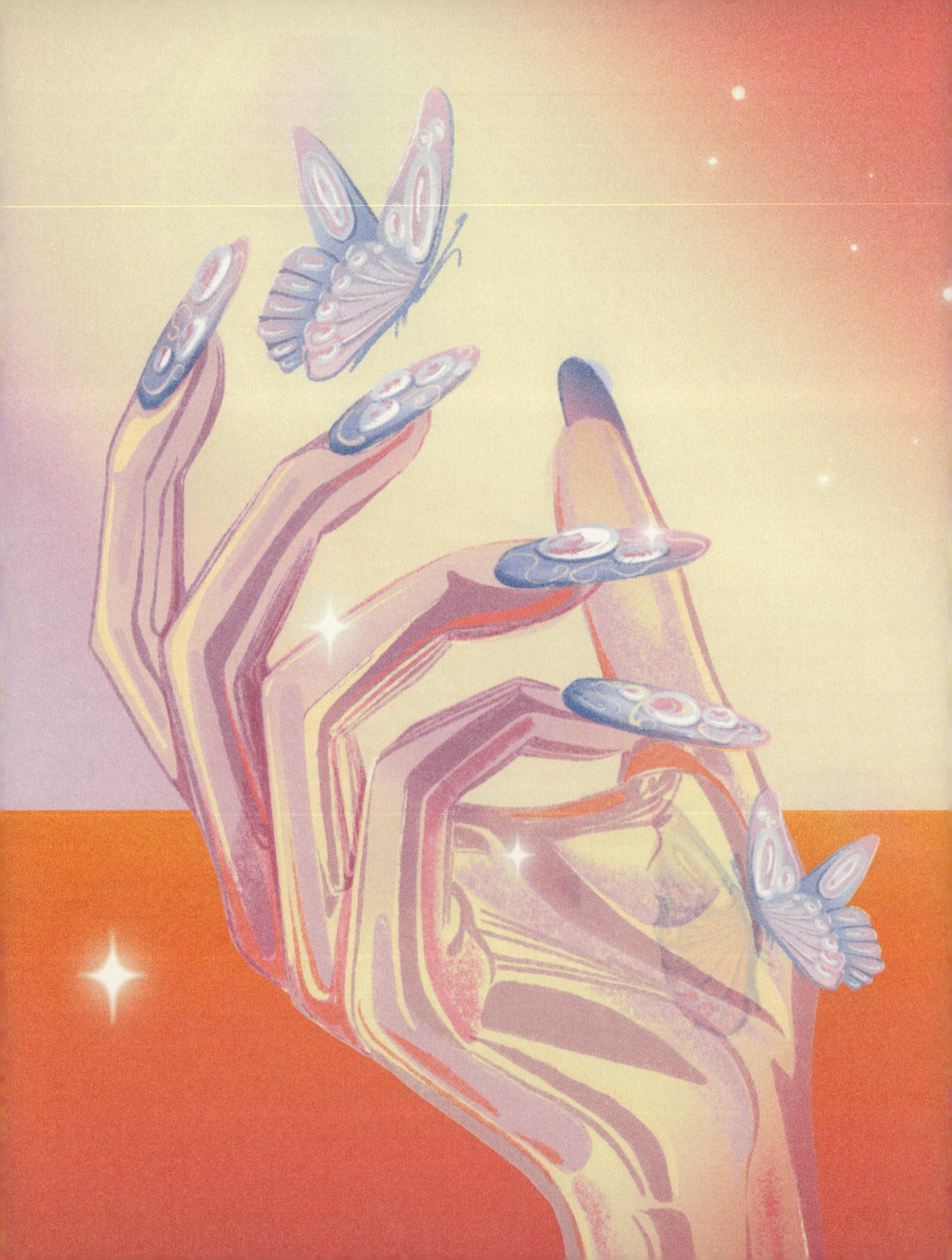

CHAPTER

NAIL ART NOW

ONE

*N*ail art has been endlessly shaped and reshaped by history, politics, nature, celebrities and technology, so there's no way one single artist could capture the vast cultural influences that make it the medium it is today. I wanted to gather voices from across the globe to answer three questions that I think are key to getting to the heart of what makes nail art such a central part of so many people's lives and daily expressions of self.

I'm lucky enough to be a part of an industry that relies heavily on the magic of connection to thrive, so it was a privilege to talk to different nail artists about their earliest memories of nail art, the moment they knew they wanted to be a nail artist and the legacy they want to leave behind. The range of answers, the way nail artists create and the community itself reflects the wider world and the rapid pace at which nail art changes. The answers are intimate, eye opening and carefully considered, much like the medium itself.

though so much to the nail artists who lent their words,
Some WORDS from the EXPERTS

Thank you so much to the nail artists who lent their words, memories and voices to give the book a broader perspective of a varied practice all centred on one shared passion.

What's your earliest memory of nail art?

KAYSIA JOY FAIR

My earliest memory of nails goes back to my childhood in the Philippines, surrounded by my mother and all my aunties. I vividly remember her beautiful natural long nails, always adorned in various shades of reds, black or sparkly pink hues.

I remember visiting my mother's province in Pampanga, there was one woman who did everyone's nails while her husband cooked and ensured everyone was well-fed while she worked her way through the line of 10 plus manicures. Despite having limited resources, they always had impeccably manicured nails and the sense of community this craft would bring always stuck with me.

To this day, my mum maintains this tradition, always keeping her nails beautifully done and it has been a cherished experience for me to be able to do her nails every month – she still loves a bold colour or classic French tip!

@SLOWER.HANDS

Toko Hutcheson

When I was seven years old, living in Tokyo at the time, I was looking through the magazines in our local conbini (convenient store) when I found a *Nail* editorial issue. I had no idea nails could look like that. It was like once I saw nail art, I couldn't unsee it. And it was everywhere, from the shop attendants, check out chicks or the hot, cool girls I was staring at on the train.

@ANGELCITYNAILS

Mutsa Evelynah Munyawiri

Hilariously and super inappropriately, my earliest memory of nail art is from when I first saw the film, *Showgirls*.

I watched it when I was really young and considering how dark it was, my main takeaway was the main character's mispronunciation of 'Versace' and the fact that she did her own nails.

I particularly remember the super glitzy black and gold nails she does at the end of the film and thinking how cool it was that she could create those designs on herself.

@MEMNAILS

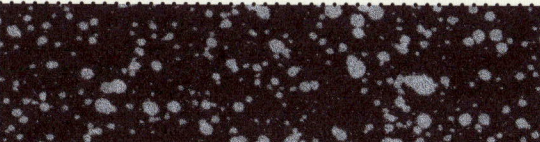

LUCAS LEVON

My earliest and still strongest vision of nail art was in Vietnam when I was 19. I was visiting my brother, and we did a road trip in the North. We stopped by a waterfall, and we saw a group of men chatting and smoking cigarettes near by the water, one of them had one hand with pink stilettos and cherry flower nail art on them. I was shocked to see such a masculine figure talking with charisma with his friends or colleagues. They really had that mafia vibe, and my brother talked to them, his wife was a nail artist, and she was practising on him.

@TEXTO_DALLAS

Sarah Elmaz

Probably my earliest memory of nail art or nail art mediums was when I was around 12 or 13 years old, and my mum had bought nail foil! It was in a little pack of three with some foil glue, and I think she used or tried to use it to add some pizazz to her nails. There really was no hand-painted nail art being done then.

Moving on a few years later, in my late teens and living in the UK, my friends and I were obsessed with long, airbrushed nails. We would travel to the only salon in Seven Sisters, London, that did that style. I would get super long nails airbrushed with palm trees and sunsets; I loved them so much. At that time, the only other type of nail art around was acrylic glitter tips, and if you had that on your nails in a regular day job, it was wild!

@GETBUFFED

TANYA BARLOW

My first memory of long painted nails is definitely from my mum and aunties long, red, shiny curved and thick talons. Through my young eyes, there was nothing more glamorous than a painted long nail. My mum and aunties never had nail art, but I do remember walking past nail salons as a child and seeing those boards full of white, black and silver swirls and flicks, rhinestones and Bauhinia flowers, two diagonal stripes in lieu of a French tip. Just, glamour, glamour, glamour!

But nail art, on myself? Visiting the hallowed halls of Wah! nails in London, 2010, I got some tuxedo nails and a moustache after daydreaming about seeing them for years and leafing through their nail art book!

@HELLOTANYA

HANH PHAM

I remember walking past a small store on Lonsdale St in Melbourne's CBD during a high school excursion. They had these adorable strawberry nails inspired by Japanese nail artists, and I became so obsessed with recreating them using nail polish. I got all the colours together and used sticky tape to make these triangle stencils for the leaves. They didn't turn out great, but that moment opened my eyes to a new form of creative expression.

@HANH.HANDS

Lili Taylor

I remember becoming aware of nails as art in films and the first I recall was *Batman Returns*. I remember seeing Michelle Pfifer, as Catwoman, creating claws out of thimbles and hooks and other things and I was obsessed with it.

I don't know when I first saw painted designs on nails, but I was more into the idea of the nails being something else; the nail looking like something other than a nail, rather than a nail with paintings on. Of course, I now also love that too, but to start with I would cello tape things to my fingers, like screws or leaves, and get lost in my own world.

@LILITAYLORNAILS

What do you want your legacy in the nail art world to be?

Isabella Rodriguez

I'd love for my legacy to be helping bridge eastern and western trends, especially crossing New York nail art with Tokyo nail art.

@SUCRE.ISA

MUTSA EVELYNAH MUNYAWIRI

Passion, mostly. I've thought about wanting to be a positive example for other brown women, girls and people who have been systematically stifled and made to think they can't express themselves freely. And to show that it's also never too late to find something you love and that loves you back.

@MEMNAILS

DONNA CAO

The legacy I want to have in the nail art world is more a mentality that this is a community where we support and inspire each other. But directly with art itself, is that you can start with what you have and where you are. It fosters a different and unique kind of creativity.

@DONNACAO

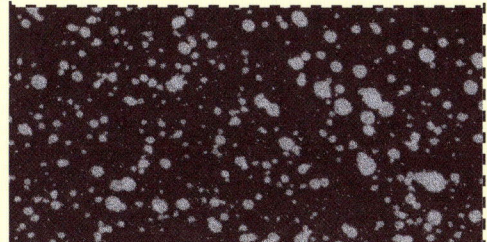

Shani Subira

I want my legacy in the world of nail art to be the standard and ethos of my practice and how I made people feel during their nail services. To provide a joy-filled experience where people can feel safe, comfortable advocating for their nail needs, create positive grooming habits and become consumed by the joy of having art on their fingertips. I want to inspire talented Black women to pursue creative and holistic beauty practices, follow their hearts and to celebrate and express themselves freely, starting with cute nails.

I would also love for my nail art to get to a place where it truly starts conversations within the beauty community around colourism, anti-Blackness, joy and holistic health.

@HAPPYHANDSNYC

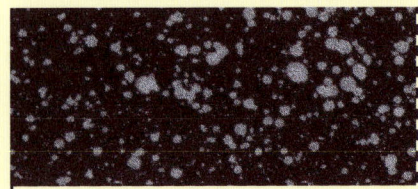

Chantel Robinson

When I first started doing nails, I wanted my legacy to be a contribution to Black culture and the beauty within it. Growing up and watching my favourite celebrities step out with glamorous looks always left me in awe; I wanted to feed my inner child by being a part of those moments. Now that I'm five years in, the legacy I desire has the same essence, but I understand the true art and complexity of what goes into nails. I want to be able to marry nails and the art world together, having my work in galleries and museums, cemented in history because of how iconic or beautiful it is. It feels like a full-circle moment for the girl who was once on the other side of the screen, and I hope it inspires people like me to dream big because it's possible.

@TELLYTALONS

LILI TAYLOR

That trans and queer people can define their own success, achieve it and become an influence in the world of nail art.

@LILITAYLORNAILS

Kaysia Joy Fair

In the world of nail art, I want my legacy to be that of an artist who created freely with a distinct sense of style, contributing to the evolution of the craft. I hope to be remembered as someone who was not only passionate about their art but also as an integral part of an amazing and supportive community.

@SLOWER.HANDS

Kumi Chantrill

On a superficial level I think I do want to be known. I want to work with the best artists in the world and be featured in the biggest magazines and musician's videos etc. because I love creating with other creatives. On a realer level I want those who knew me to know how much I loved my job. If I can achieve anything at all I just want to keep loving what I do.

@NAILSBYKUMI

LUCAS LEVON

My deepest purpose in nail art is to bring it to the male audience, to break the frontier that says 'nails are feminine'.

@TEXTO_DALLAS

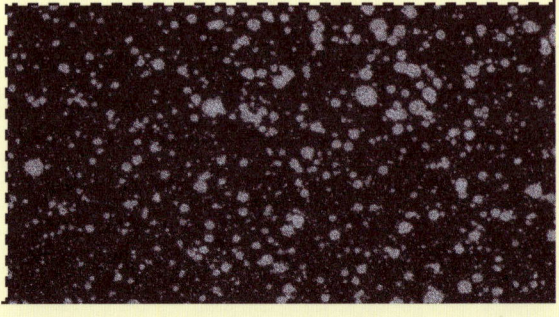

Nathan Taylor

In my journey as a nail artist, I aspire to leave a legacy that transcends mere aesthetics and speaks profoundly of advocacy, inspiration and innovation. My vision for my legacy in the world of nail art is to create a lasting impact that champions inclusion, drives transformative change within the industry and continuously pushes the boundaries of what is considered nail art today.

@BUFFBARBRISTOL

CLARA HWANG

I want people to see that doing nails as a career doesn't equate to having a dead end job. It is an incredibly dynamic career that has evolved immensely over the years and that one is well and truly capable of supporting themselves and their families doing 'just nails'. That's my personal experience having been brought up in a conservative, academic driven society that views doing nails as menial jobs. I went against the grain of the society I grew up in and ignored much naysaying about my career choice. My nail career has opened up countless doors for me, something I doubt I would have experienced had I stuck to a traditional career path. I would like people to feel empowered when they look at my work history and know that they can absolutely achieve that for themselves.

@CLARAHNAILS

LYNDA TAING

I believe that my legacy in the nail art world would be my versatility. I've never been someone to stick to one style, very much like my own personal style – a chameleon. Over the years I've met so many different characters and personalities and none of them have fit into one box. So, my goal is to fit into everyone's boxes – know every style and technique, keep pushing my limits and boundaries and be able to look back on my work and say, 'hell yeah, I did that!'.

@MANICANDIE

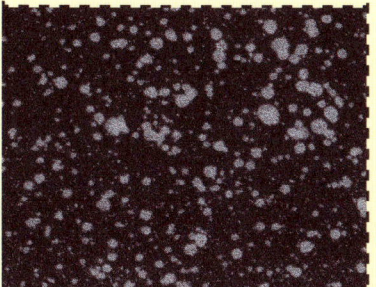

Chloe-Elizabeth Reed

I want my legacy in the world of nail art to be remembered as one of continuous learning and education. I believe that knowledge is the foundation for building better businesses. My goal has always been to educate myself and others, so we can all create more art and achieve greater financial success.

@GLAMNAILZ210

What was the moment you knew you wanted to be a nail artist?

Pria Bhamra

I started doing nail art when I was older – on myself – and it began to be more of a thing in the UK – I love drawing and illustration, so this was just another opportunity for me to paint.

@BHAMBNAILS

Yuri Osuka

I studied graphic design after high school and moved to NYC to learn more in the field. I never even went to a nail salon or got my nails done at the time, but when I saw Eichi Matsunaga's nail art, I immediately knew this is what I wanted to do. Eichi is a legendary nail artist who has been a pioneer in the industry for years. After being inspired by his work, I quit studying graphic design and started going to nail school.

@YURIOSUKA123

Mutsa Evelynah Munyawiri

For the first couple of years, I was mostly just trying stuff and didn't really know if I wanted to do it long-term. Whereas now, I feel like there's far more intention in my work and beyond content creating, I want to continue creating nail art for as long as I'm alive. Even if it's just for me.

@MEMNAILS

Shani Subira

I've been a nail enthusiast most of my life and I always knew I was good at doing nail art, but it wasn't until I met a talented Black nail artist working at a chic nail salon in Brooklyn that I saw myself working in the industry. I sought her out because not only was she a talented artist, but she was an advocate for natural nail health which is something I heavily identify with. After experiencing a nail service with her and talking with her about her journey I knew I wanted to become a professional myself and provide the same integrity-filled experience.

@HAPPYHANDSNYC

Asia Bloodworth

I think once I got exposure to more of the artistry of nails, that's when I made the decision to become a nail artist. I first got into nails and doing nail art when I was 14 years old. I looked up to different nail artists such as Viv Simmonds, Catherine Wong and Sam Biddle, who were the top award-winning nail artists in the world during the time I was getting started with my nail artist journey, and I had the chance of interviewing them on my podcast, *Nails and Beauty Talk.*

@ASIATHABIRD

Chloe-Elizabeth Reed

Growing up in Detroit, MI during the 80s, I was surrounded by a vibrant mix of styles and techniques. It was the height of Detroit's industrial boom, with GM, FORD and Chrysler dominating the scene. This prosperity fuelled artistic expression in every aspect of life. My aunts were always sporting beautifully designed nails, both long and short, with intricate designs on every single finger. I vividly remember thinking, 'I'm going to do that one day!' That early exposure ignited my passion for nail art, setting me on the path I'm on today.

@GLAMNAILZ210

Maria Salandra

My mother's nail tech was amazing she didn't even speak English, she was Cuban and the most beautiful woman, we managed to communicate with each other. I knew then, at age 10, when she taught me how to do a nail extension with waxing muslin.

@REDHOTNAILS

Claudia Spirou

I automatically thought of nail artists as being tied to more traditional salons, but being exposed to solo nail techs on Instagram made me realise it could be a really intimate, personal service and you could build a unique brand image outside the traditional salon model, which made it feel like something I could pursue.

@SETSBYONYX

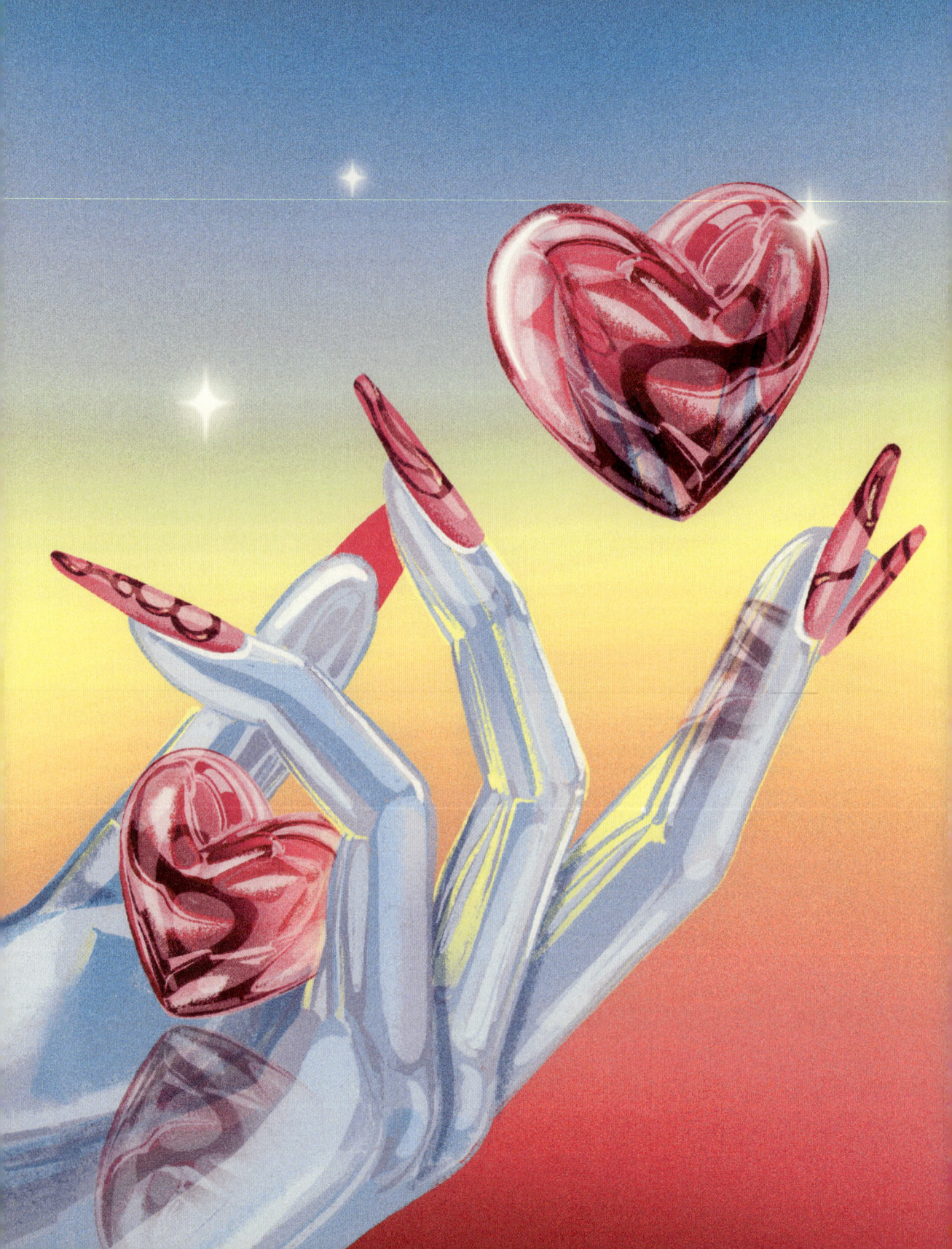

CHAPTER

MANNEQUIN HANDS SETS

TWO

A note from the author

My earliest memory of nail art dates back to the first issue of *Sabrina's Secrets*. A beauty-based magazine where *Sabrina the Teenage Witch* would give you her tips and tricks for achieving the hottest 90's hair, make-up and nail looks. Issue 1 kicked off with a nail art pen in a pearly silver hue. Those pens were clogged and congealed within the first hour of use, but the tips and tricks on how to achieve flower patterns using toothpicks were eternal.

It could've been the first dot of the silver nail art pen that started off the obsession that would ultimately render my university degree useless and make my migrant grandparents fret. Maybe it was the mysticism and intimacy of women holding hands at home when my mama and aunty would get their nails done by a mobile nail technician. Whatever started it, my love for nail art grew to be trialled and tested on myself and my very patient friends.

Eventually a talented stylist friend of mine asked if I would make nails for a shoot he was working on. I started an Instagram account to post my first editorial and pitched names to my friends. I don't remember the exact moment it clicked, but something popped into my head, a memory from the early internet. There was one on a WordPress blog where a nail artist, Sophy Robson, talked about finding a nude nail polish so well matched to your natural skin tone that your hand would achieve a mannequin hand's appearance. Not a nude nail lover myself, but someone looking for a name, it stuck.

So, Mannequin Hands was born. I left my life in marketing to pursue a life of cleaning up cuticles and I love it. It may have taken me a few years to set out a real business plan but when I got to my vision statement – a sharp one liner that's meant to sum up the entirety of what you hope to achieve in your business – I realised that my aim was to bring nail art to as many hands as possible. Now, with two hands and a little back pain, I give you this book. It's a dedication to my love of nail art and hopefully a guide of sorts, with all the basics and a little inspiration to make nail art an extension of you.

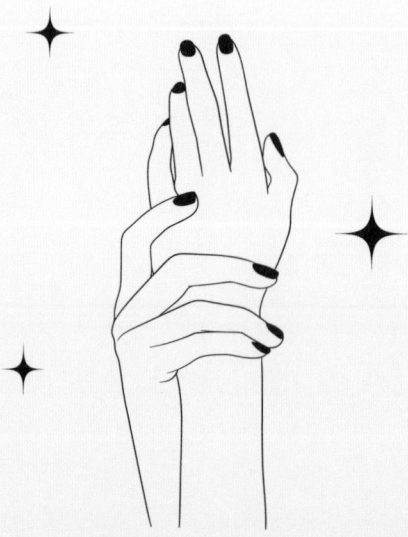

THE SETS

Inspiration for nail art can come from anywhere and anything. There are endless ways to interpret an artwork, a plant, an outfit, a movie poster, truly anything at all and bring it to life on a set of nails. Sometimes people want a literal interpretation of something, other times they're looking to use their inspiration as a jumping off point, something that emulates the essence of the inspiration rather than a tiny visual photocopy of it.

Every nail artist has a different starting point, some consider colour first, letting the colour wheel decide their next move, others layer by texture, by sculpting or giving dimension to a set using 3D gels, gems, chains and the like, while others plan out their sets to play with a new technique they've learned and expand their repertoire.

For me personally, I love a little variation. After over 10 years going one-to-one with my nail lamp, I've loved picking up new techniques along my nail journey. The constant need for variation has had me learning to work with new mediums and employing all sorts of techniques to achieve the looks my brain wants to see on my hands.

These sets are looks I loved creating, sets I made with various bits of inspiration in mind. Some of the sets started off as an imagining of what I'd love to shoot most, elements that are deeply impractical for a client, but I needed to have on a nail, nonetheless. Some sets reflect the art, fashion, nature and food I saw while ideating for this book while others were born from a desperate need to try out a new product or technique. Colour palette, texture, technique or shape informed each look and there's a memory, photo or song that I could pin to each of them.

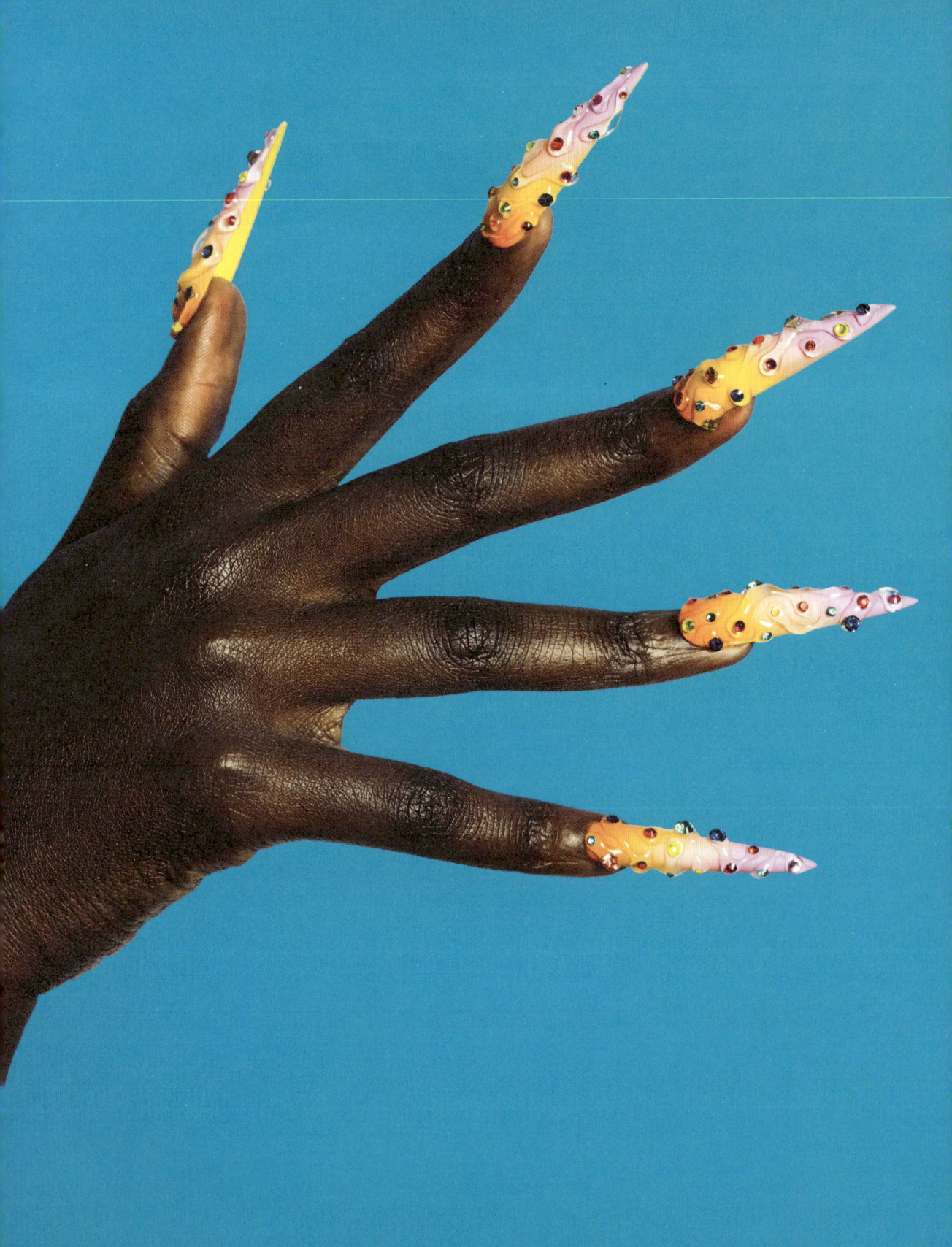

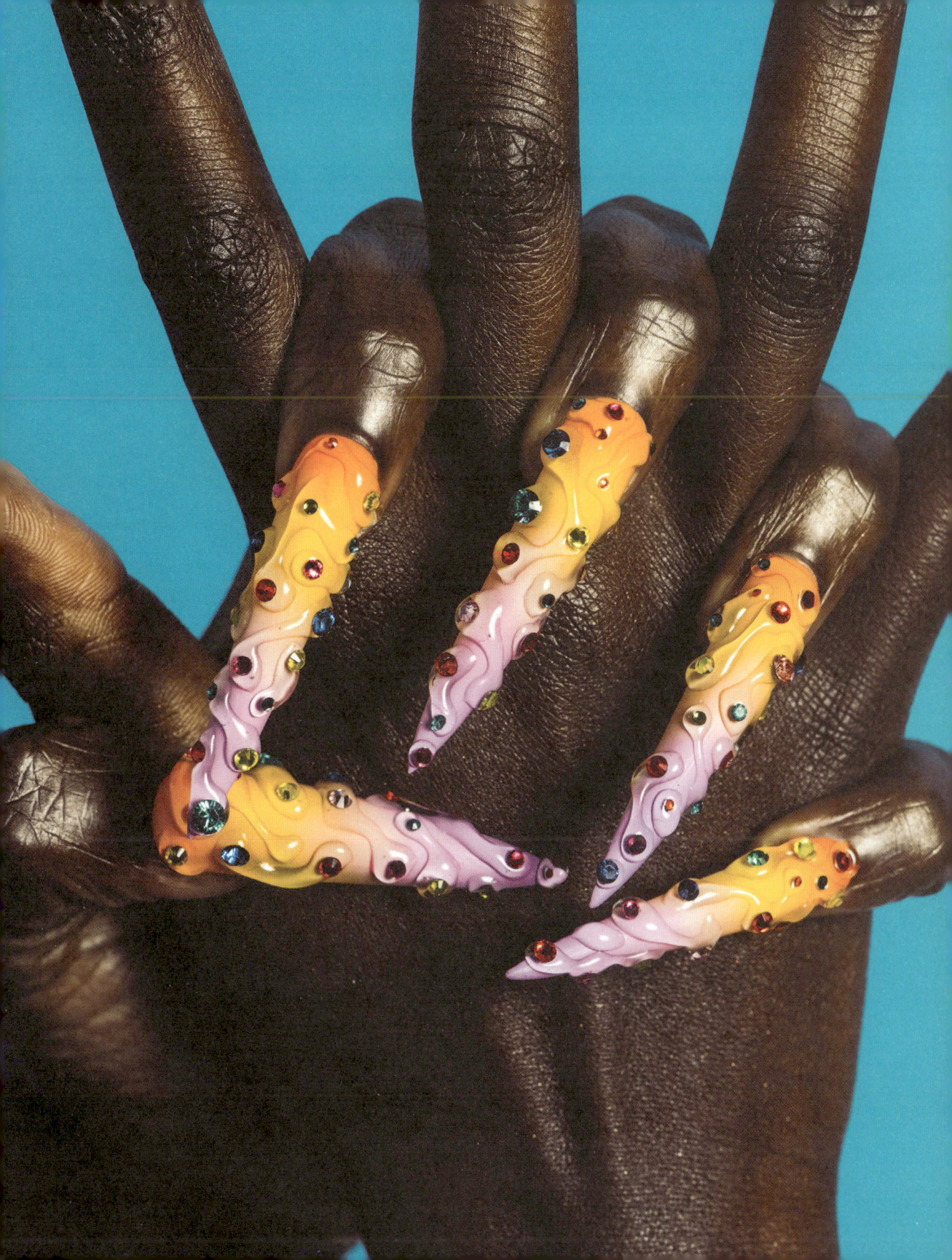

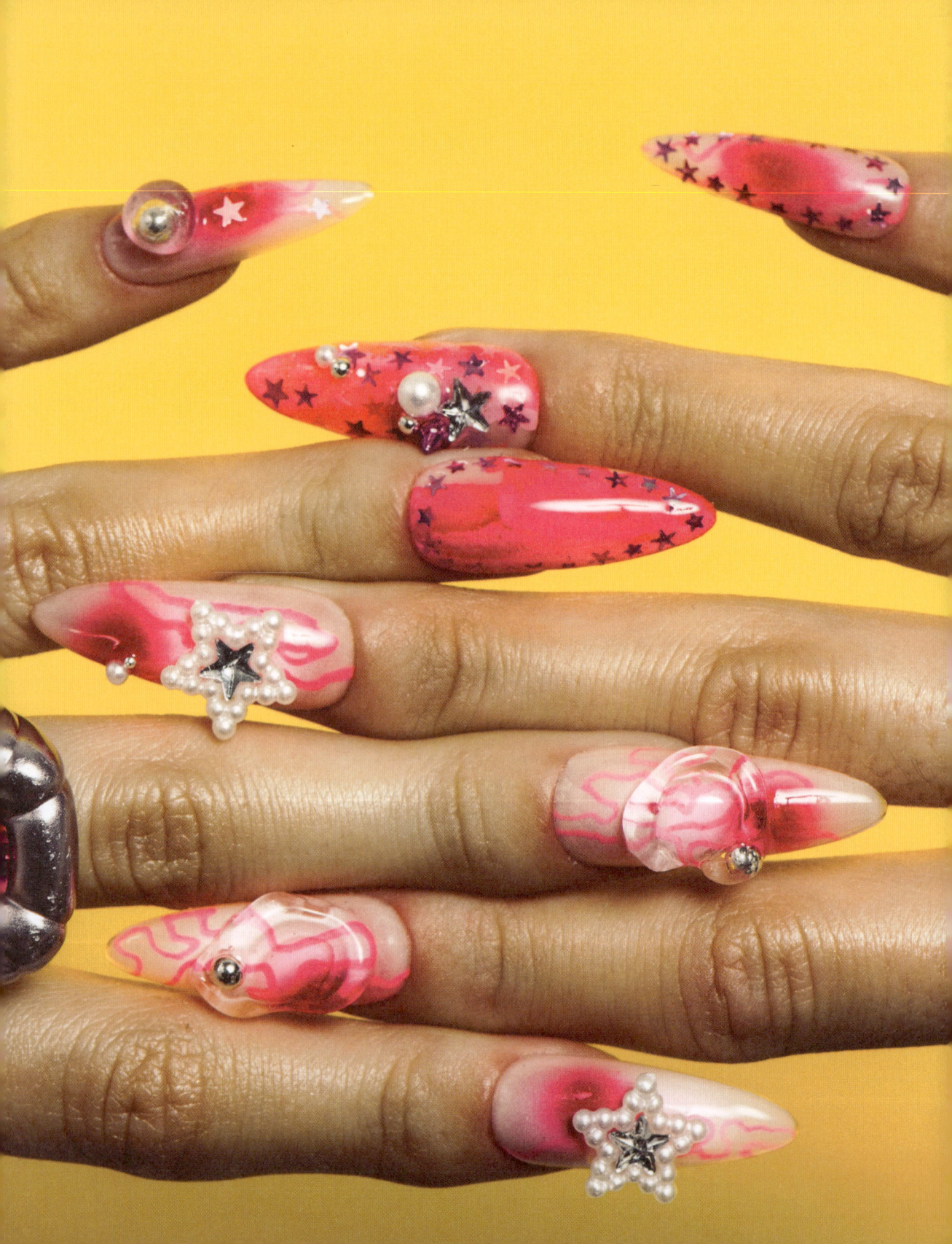

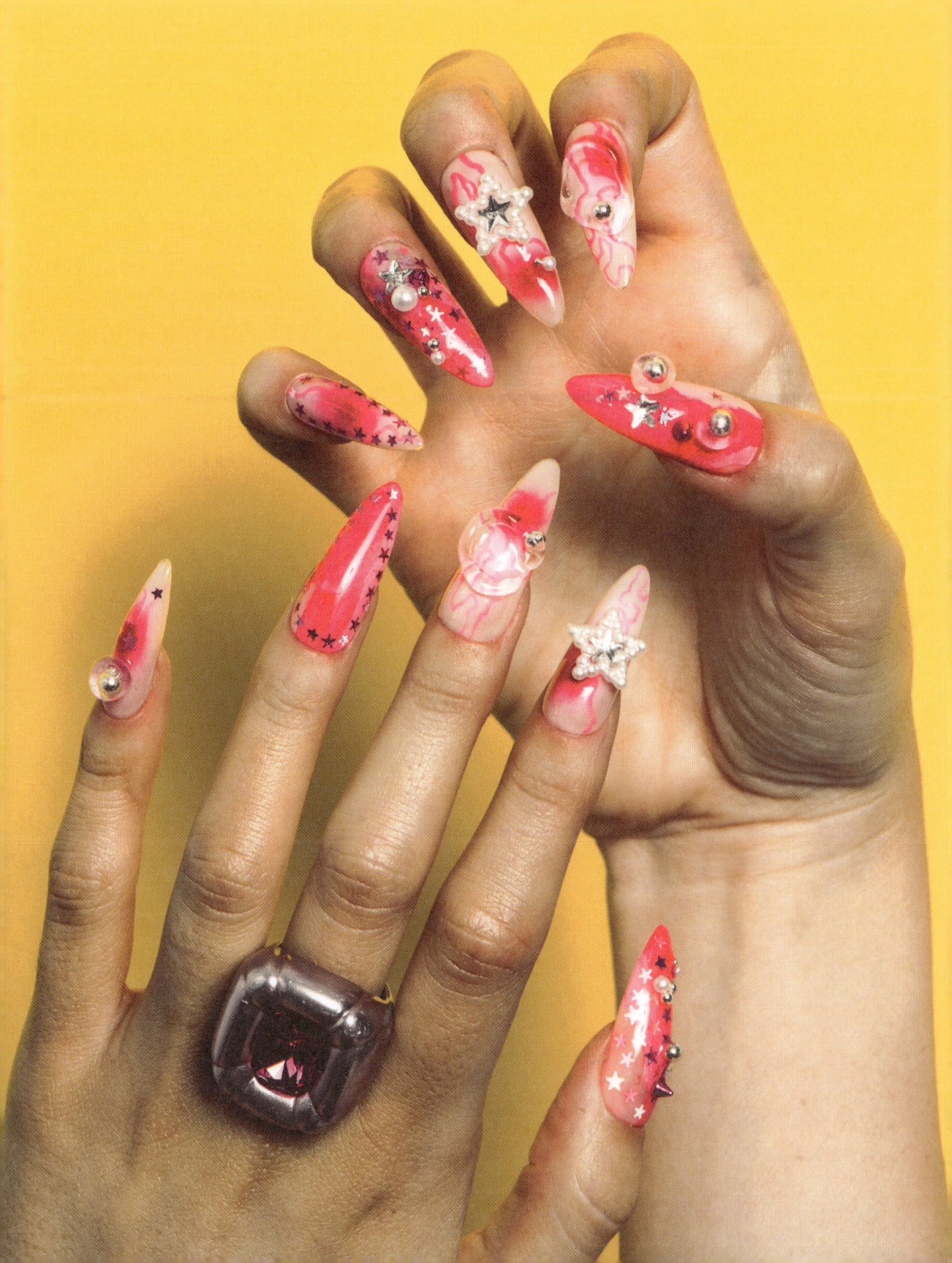

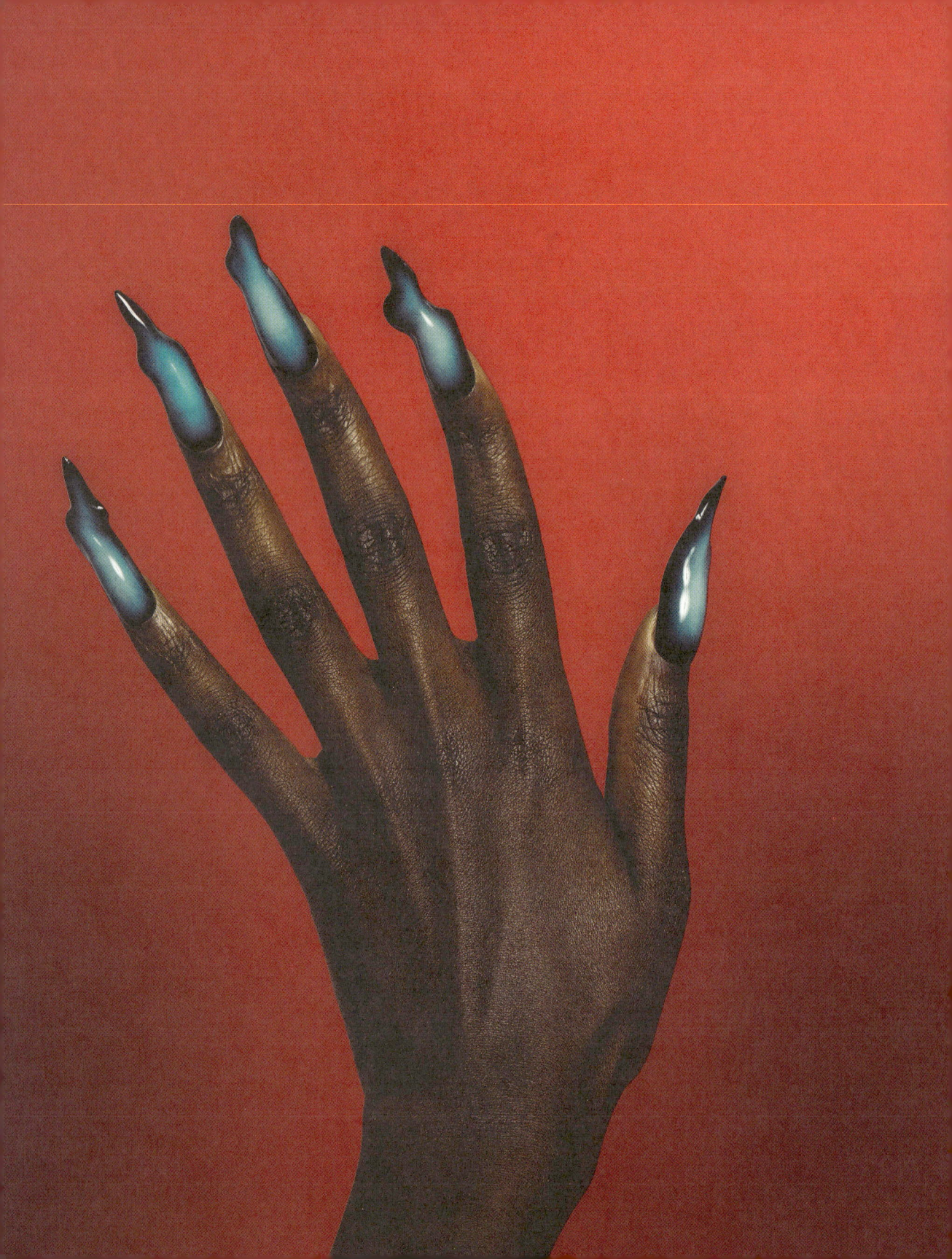

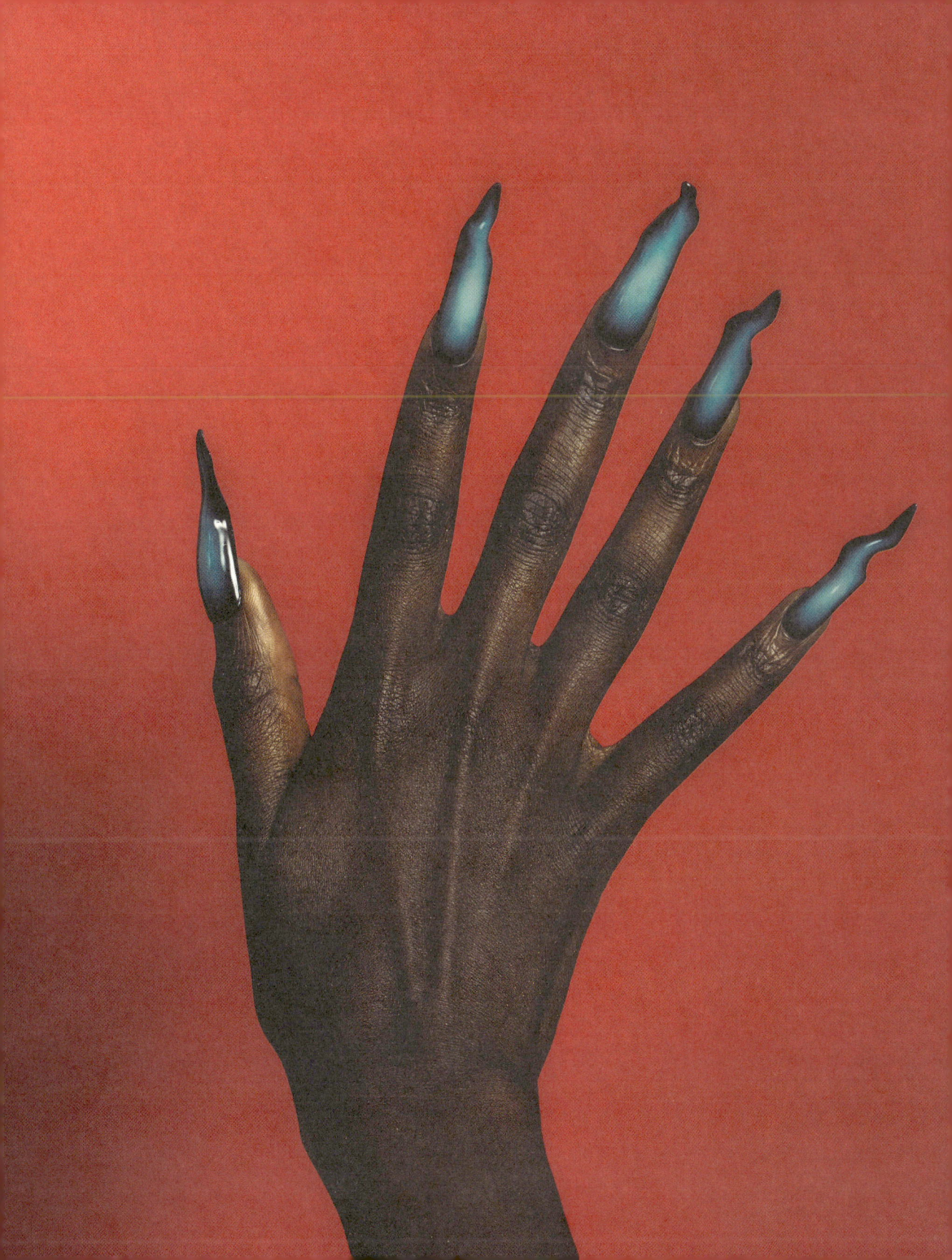

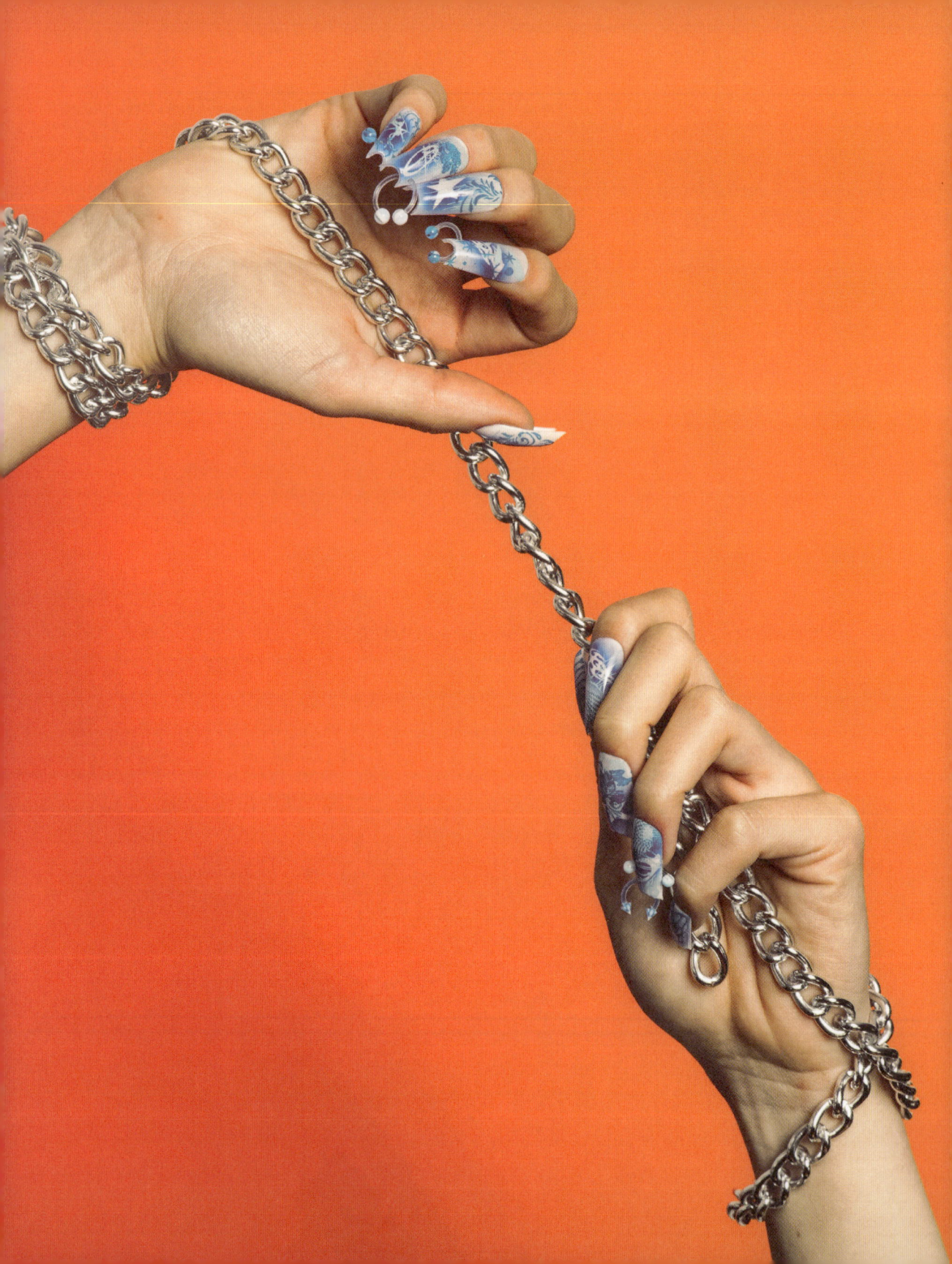

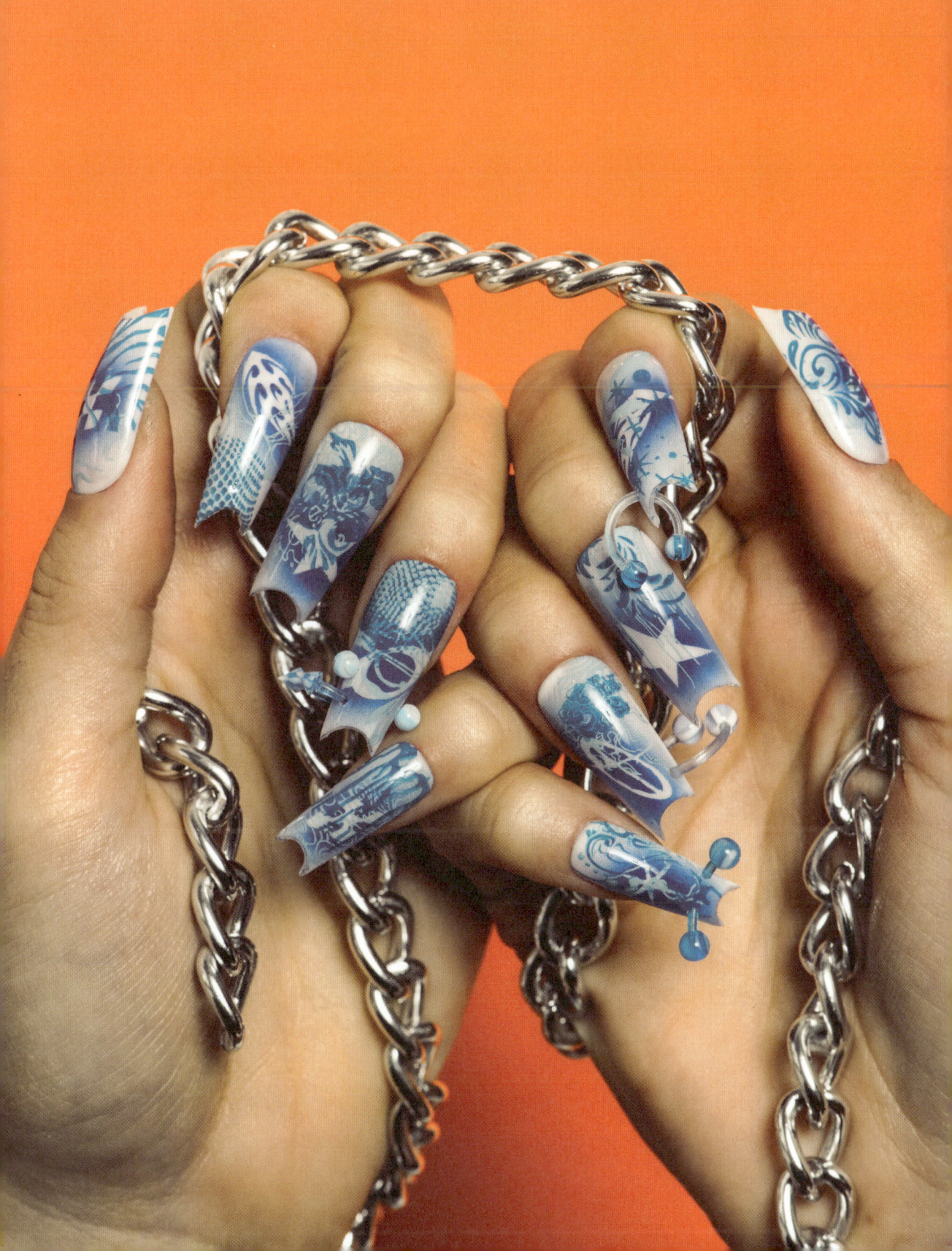

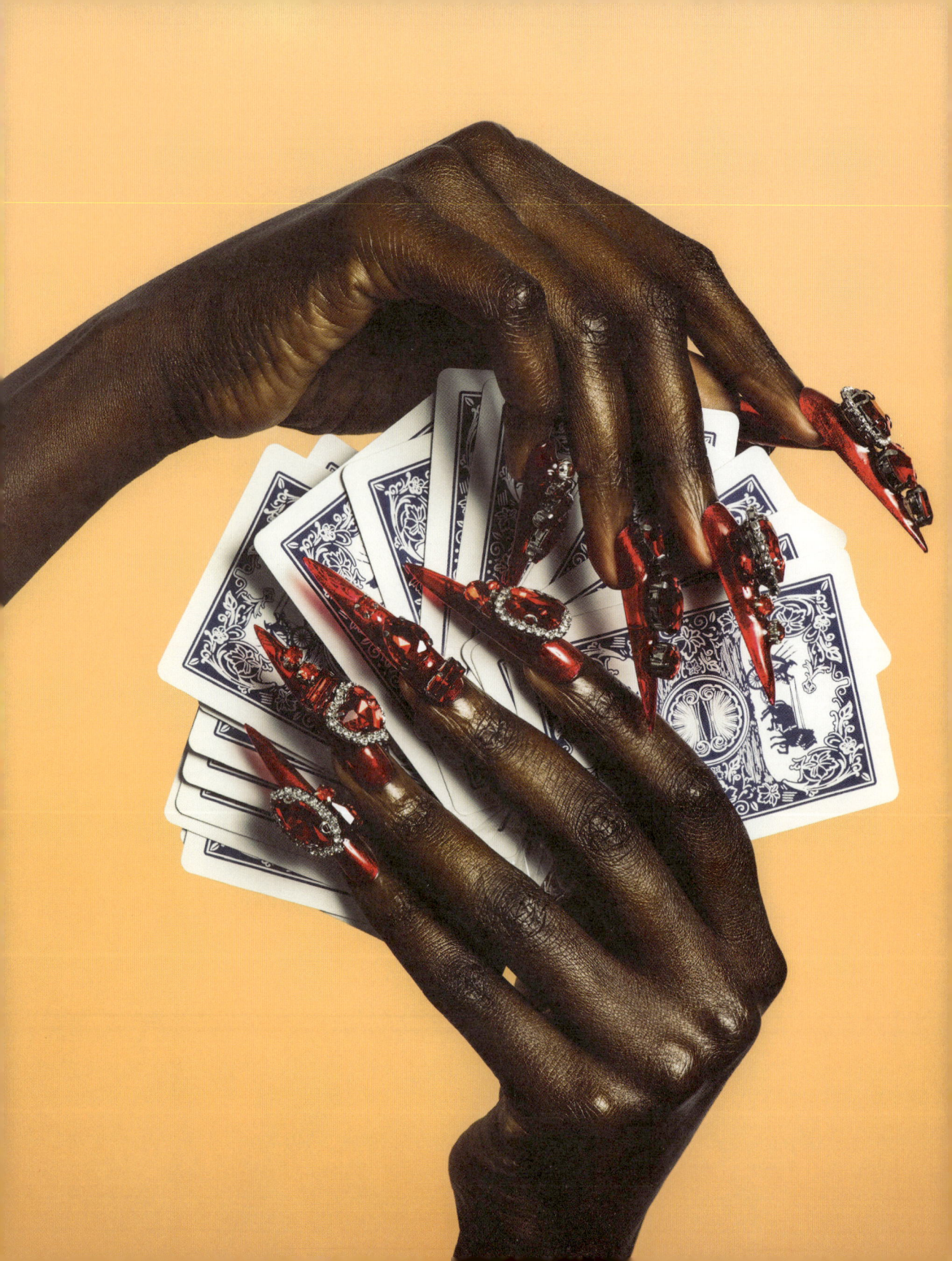

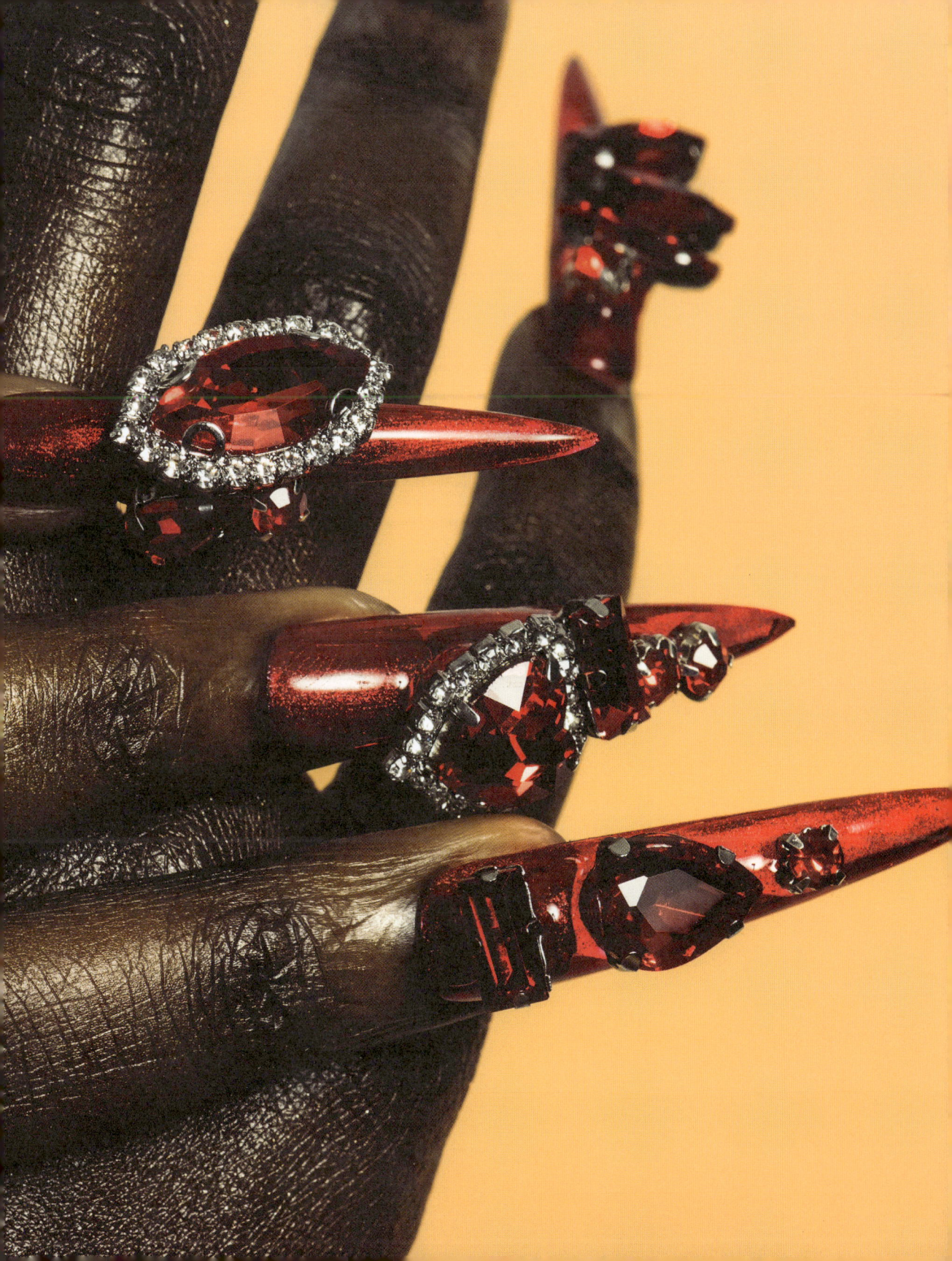

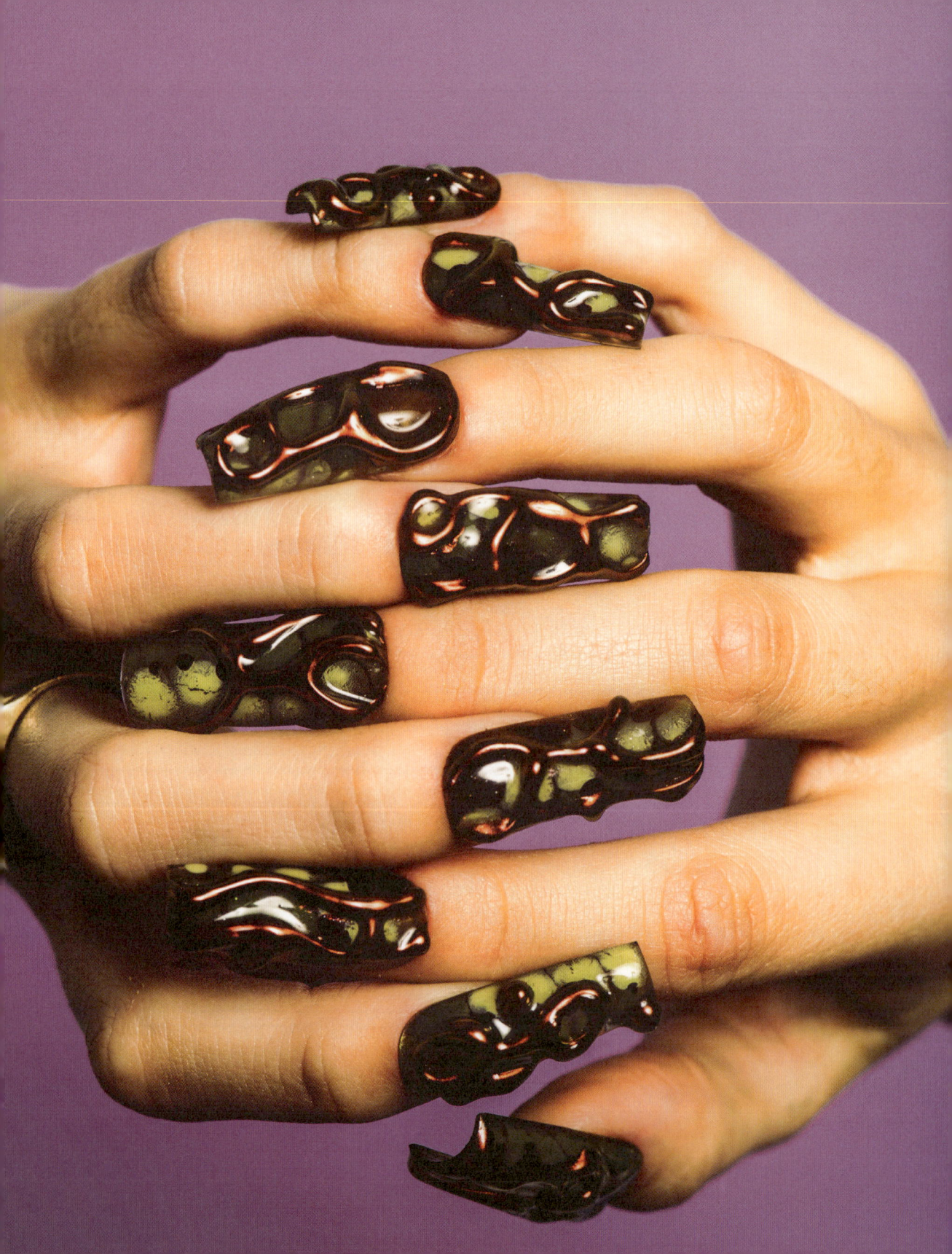

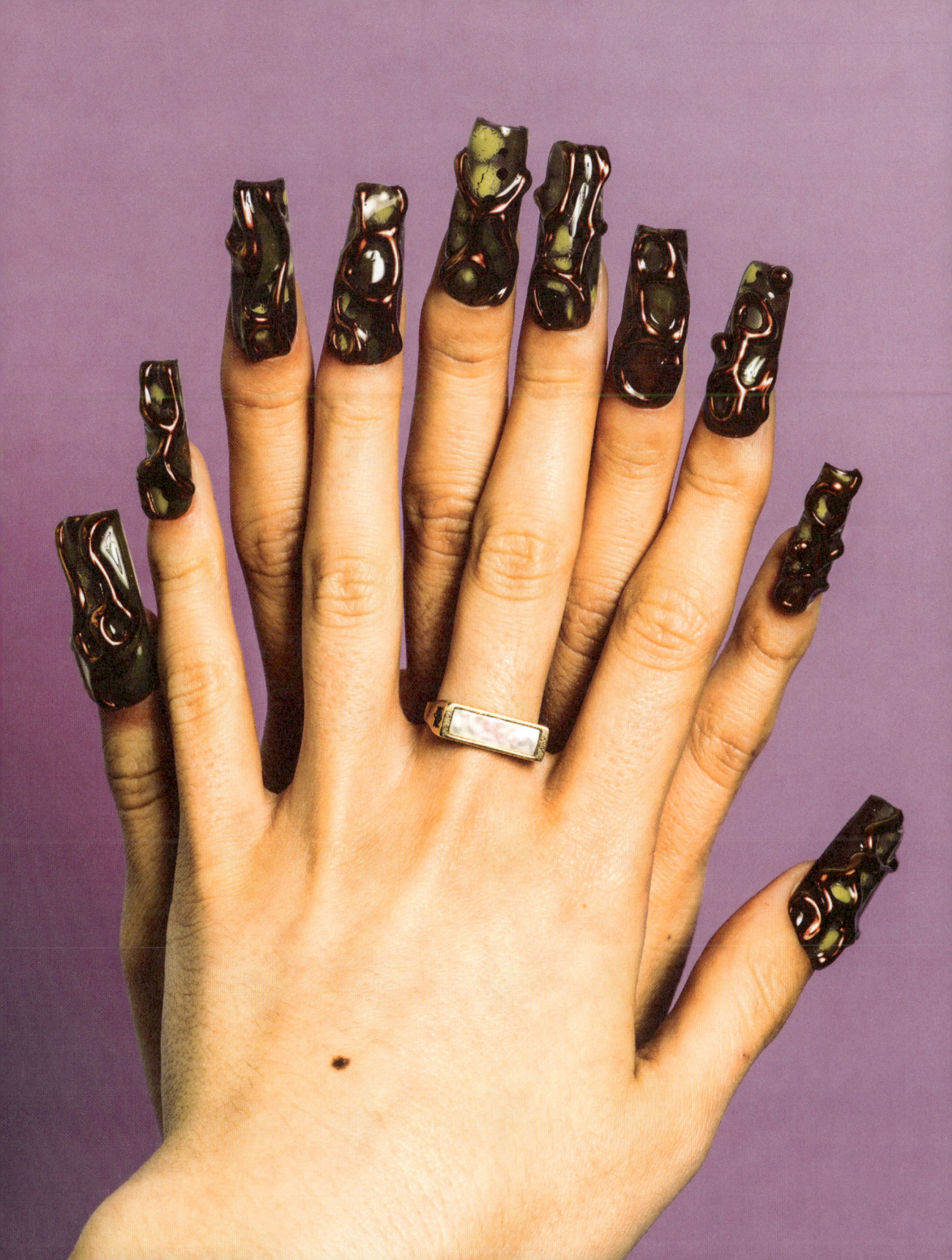

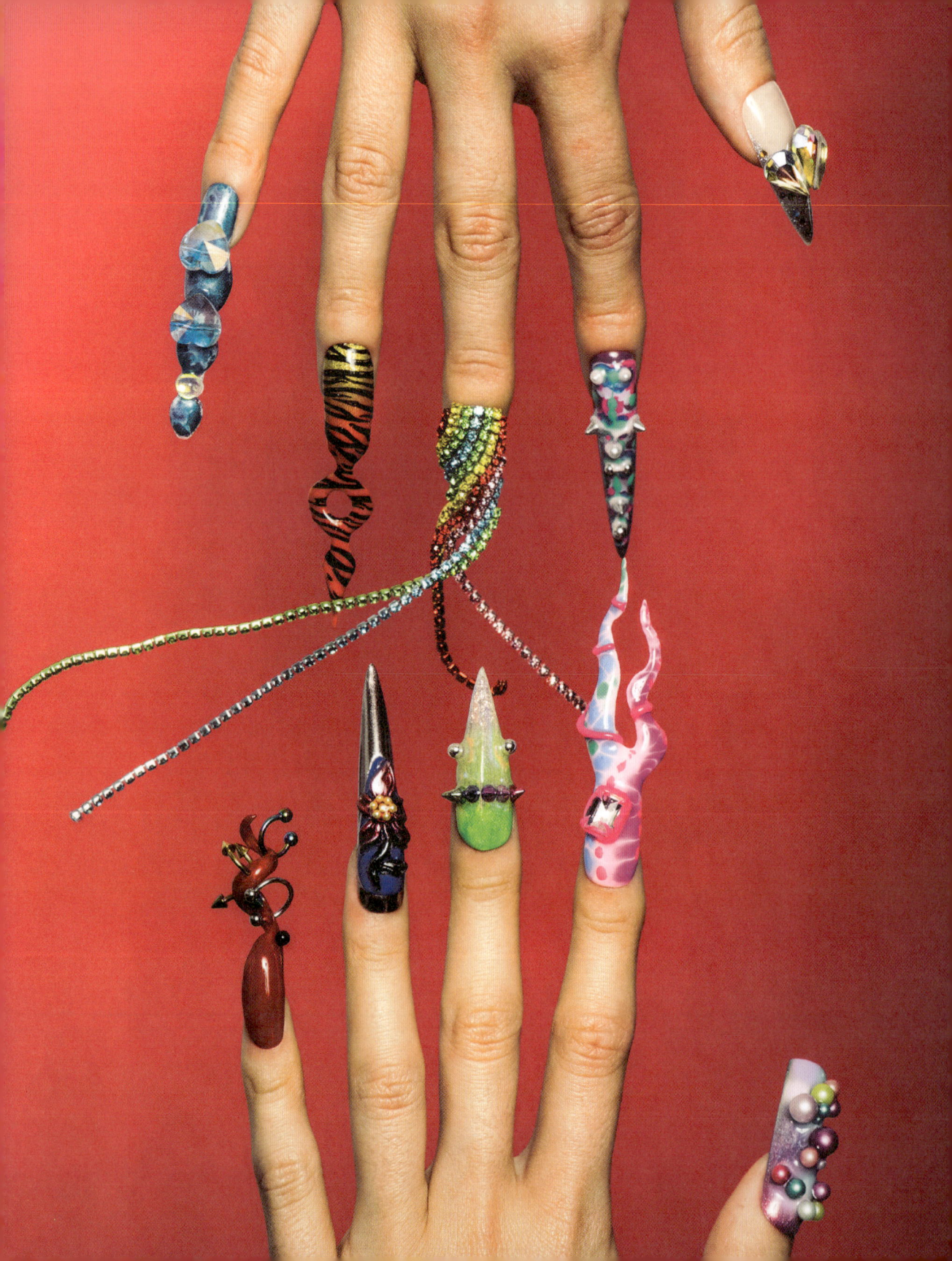

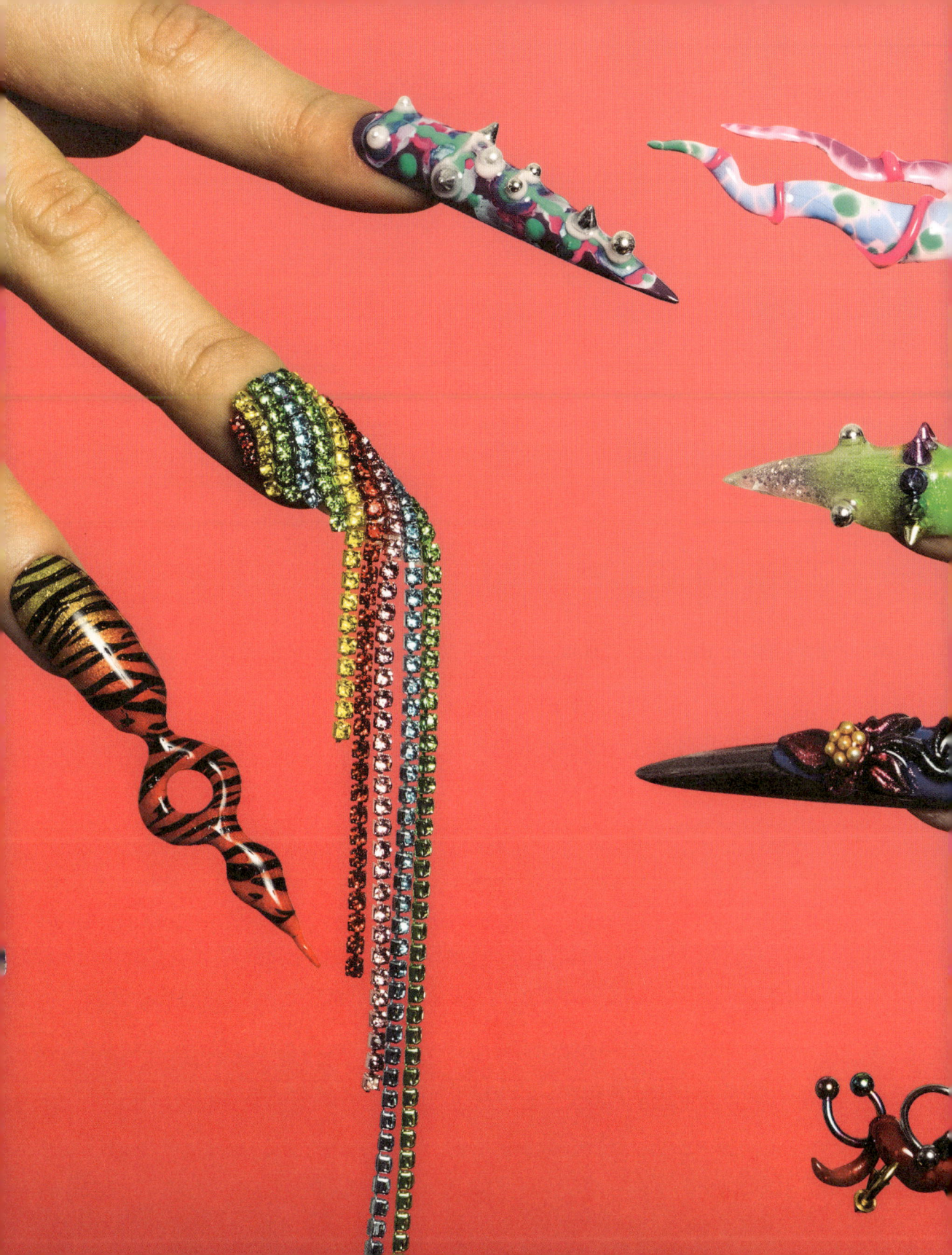

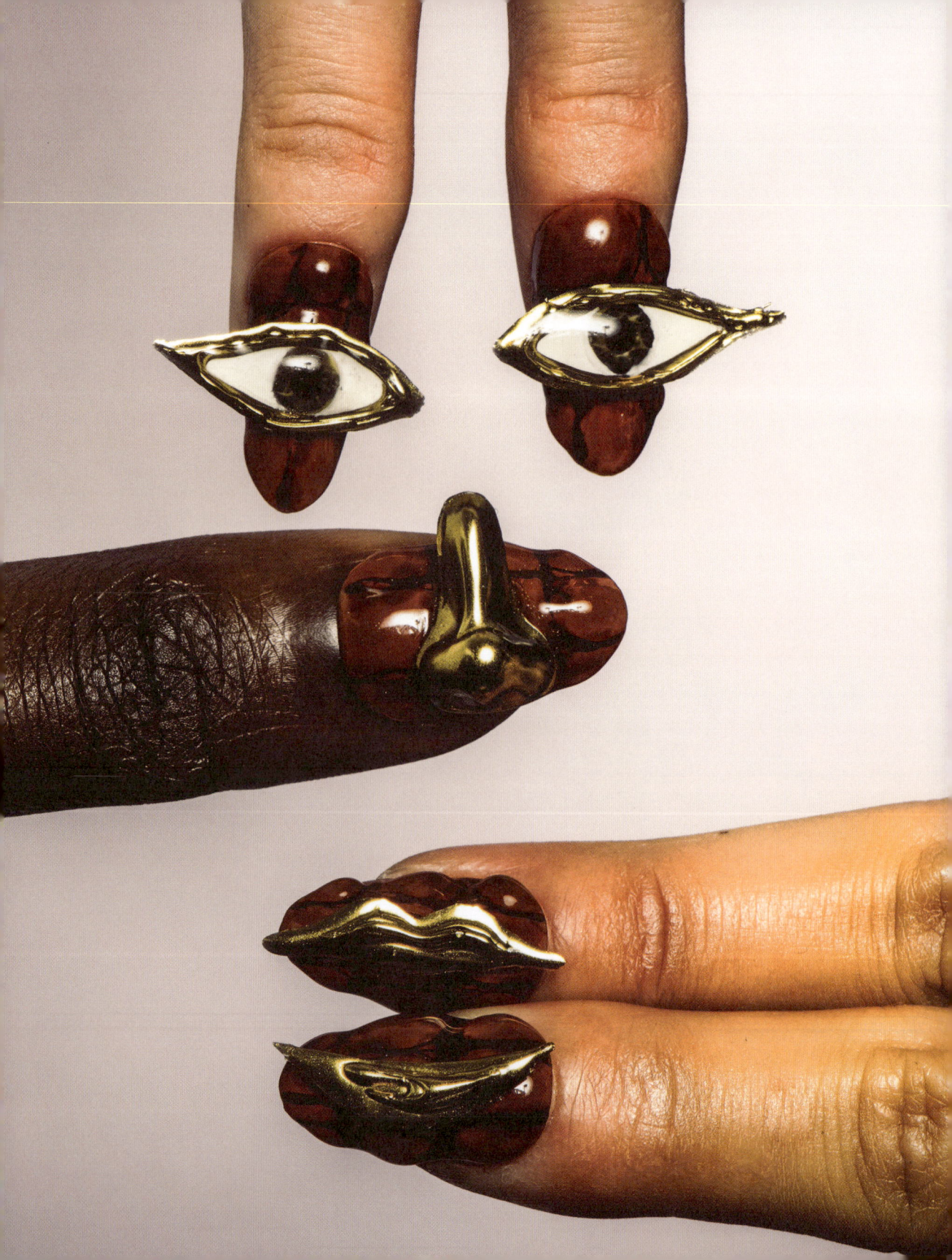

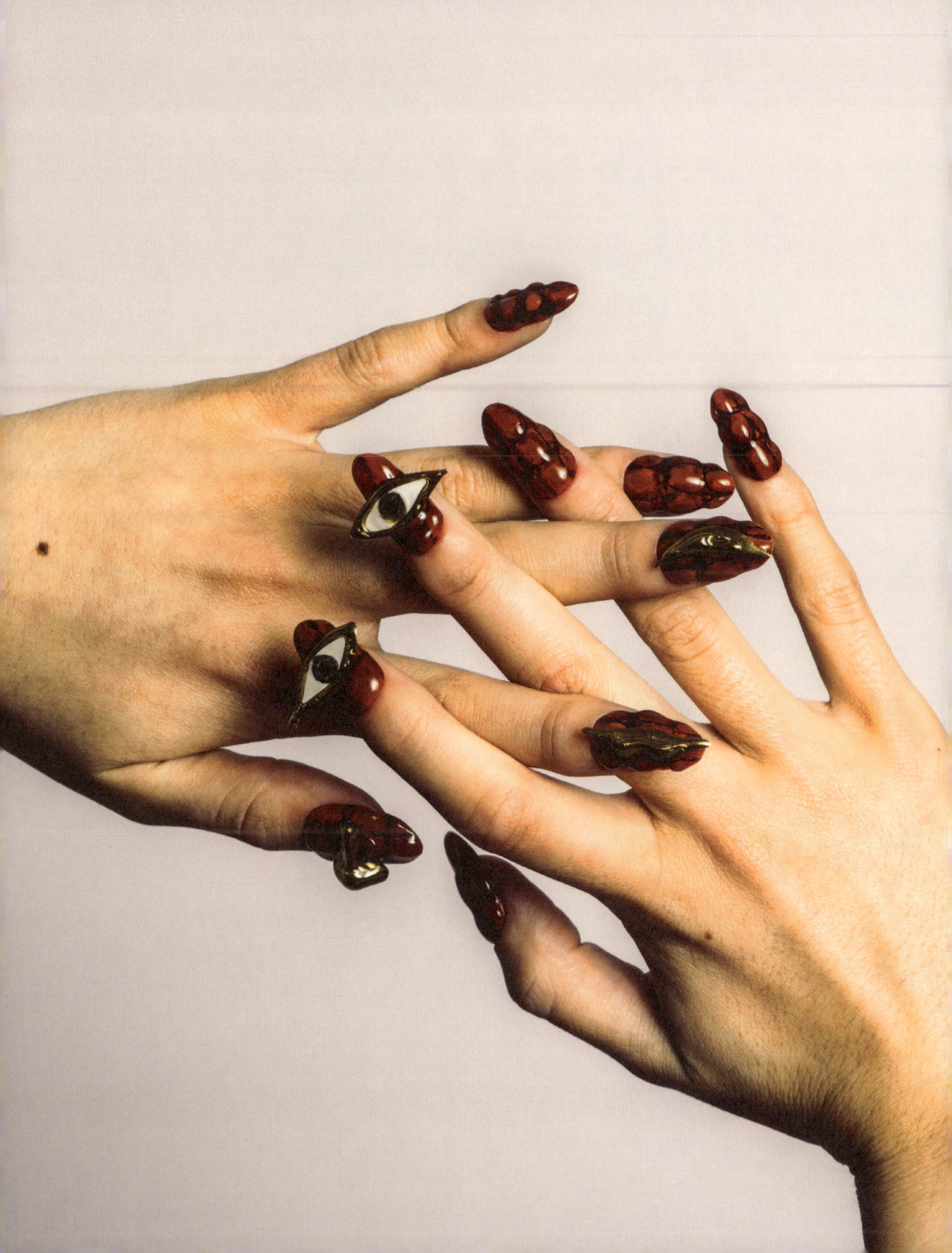

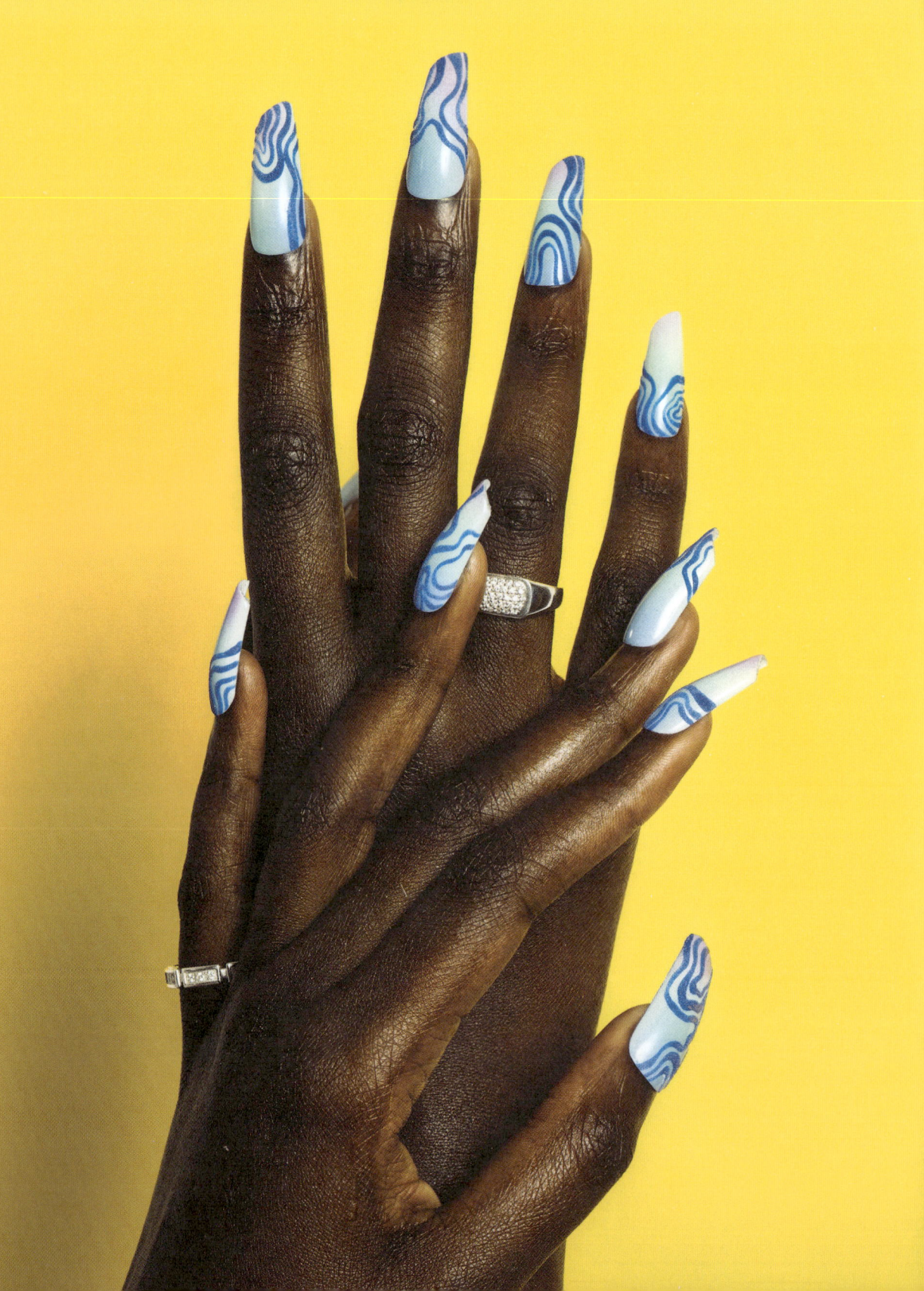

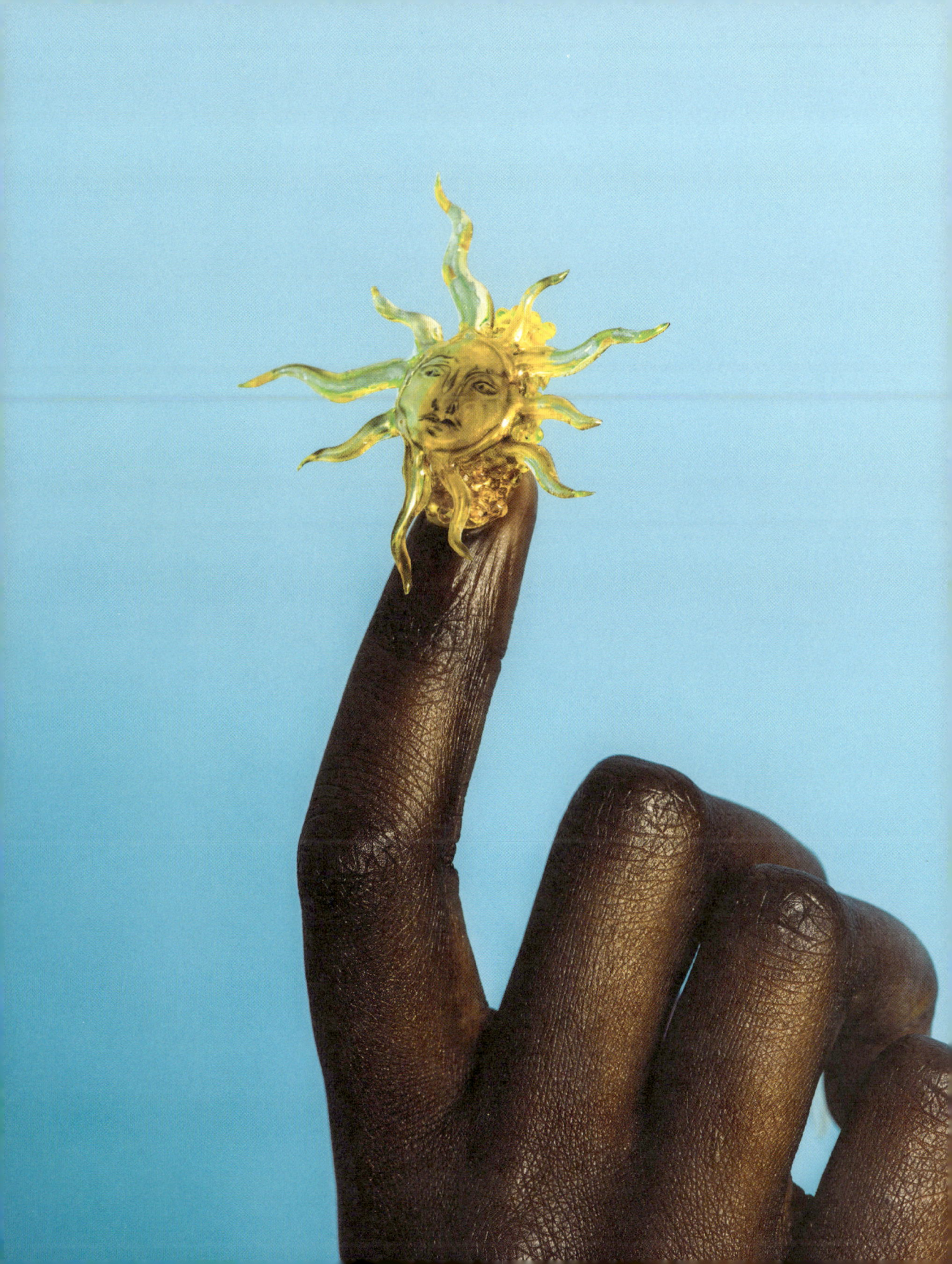

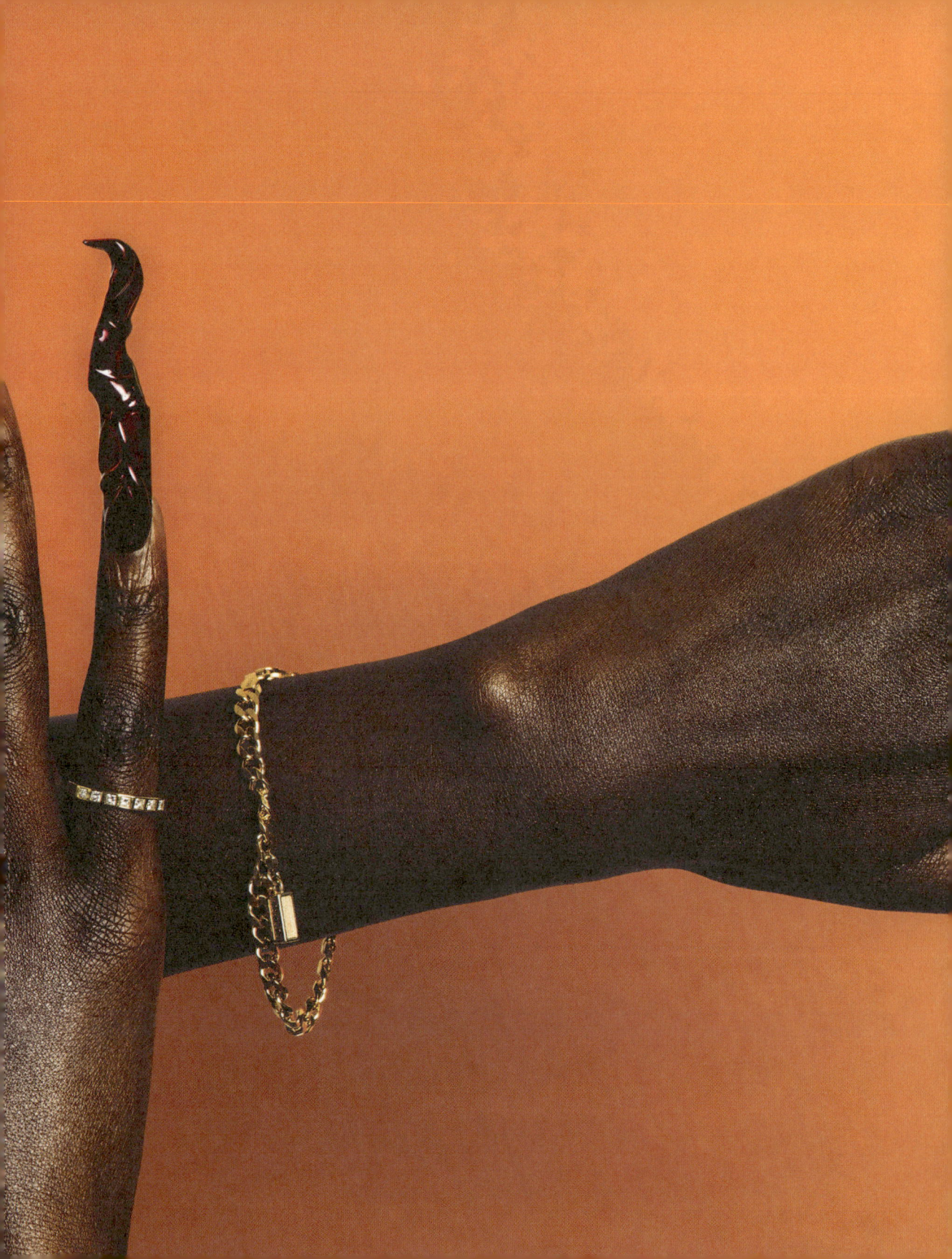

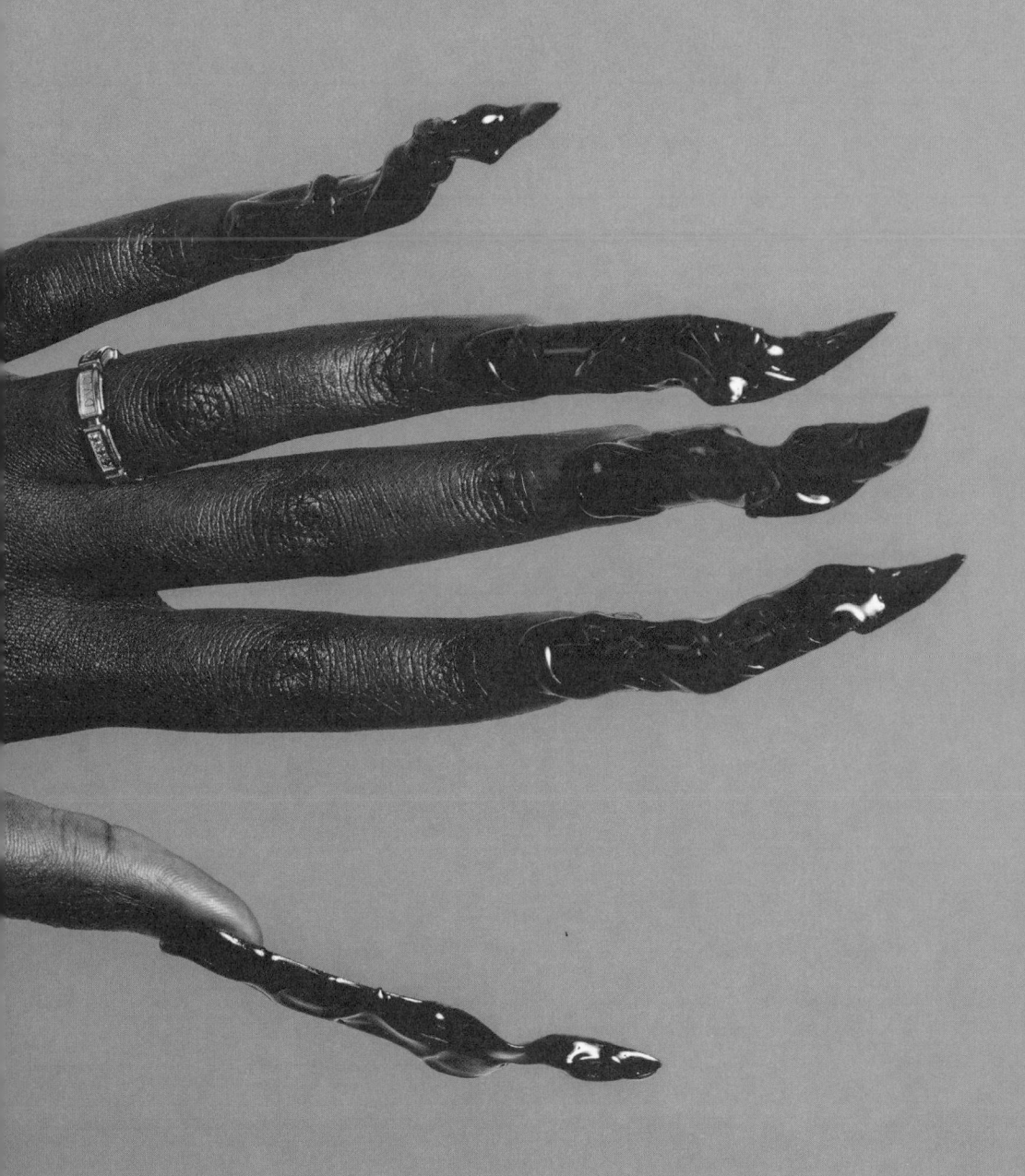

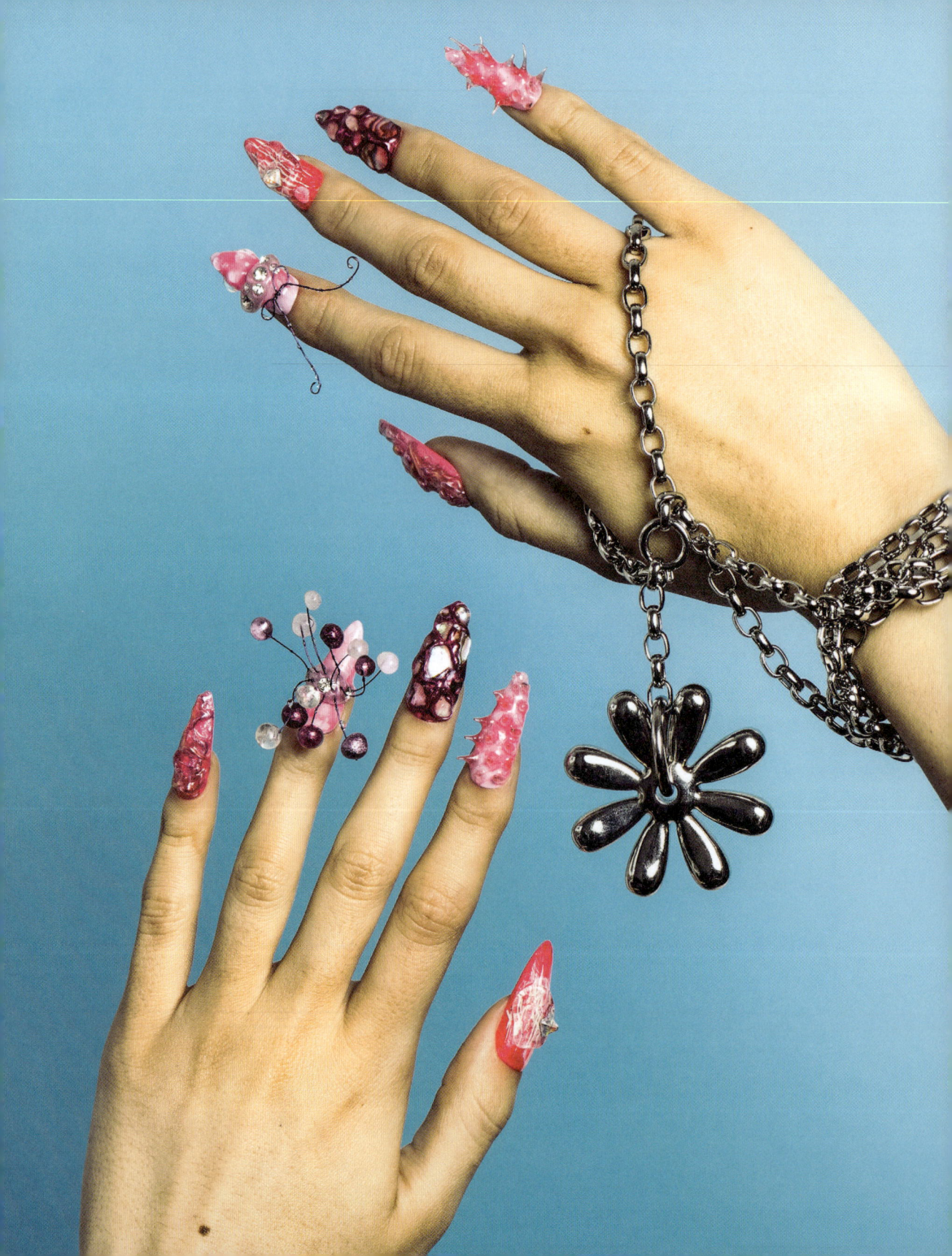

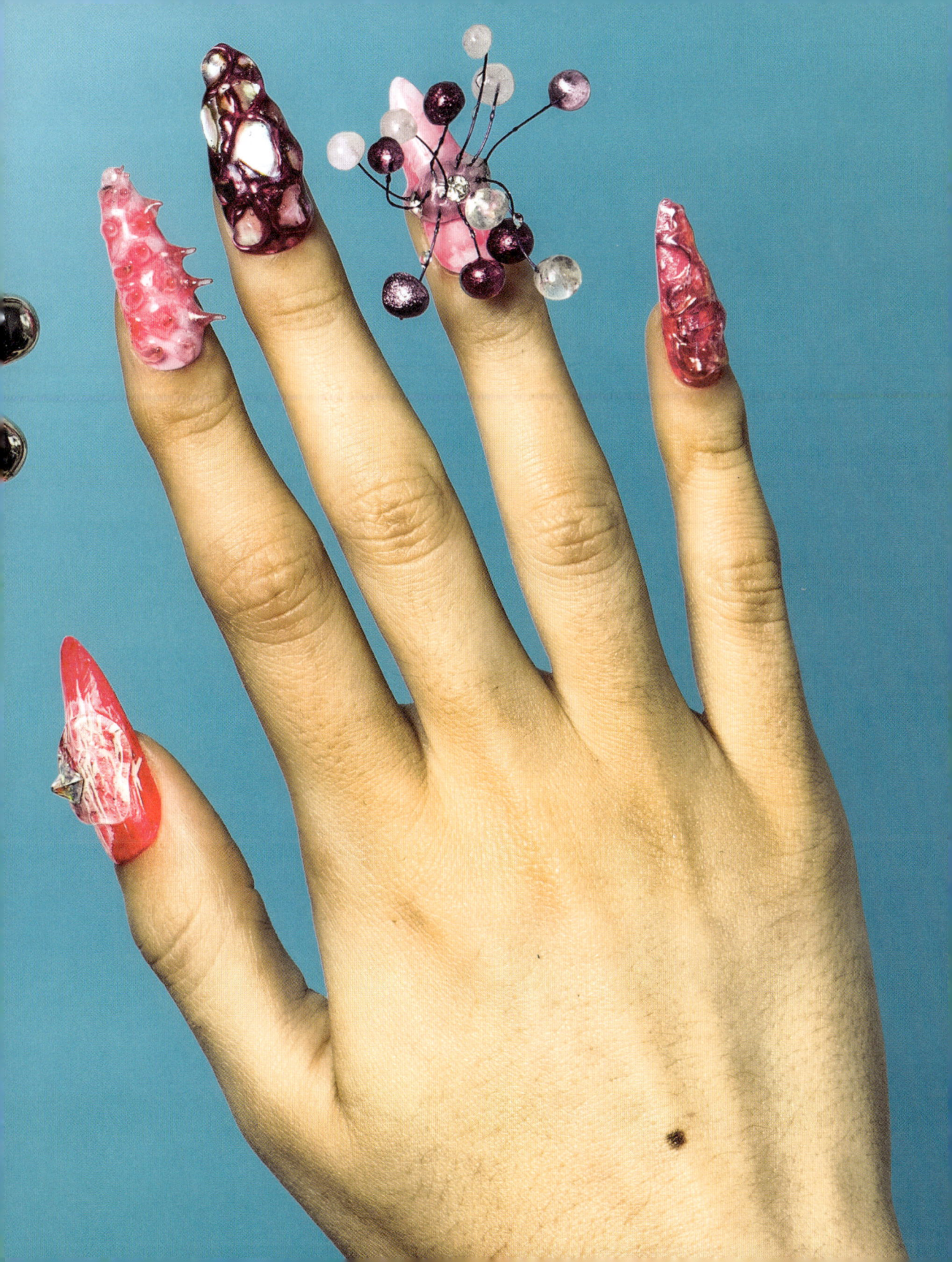

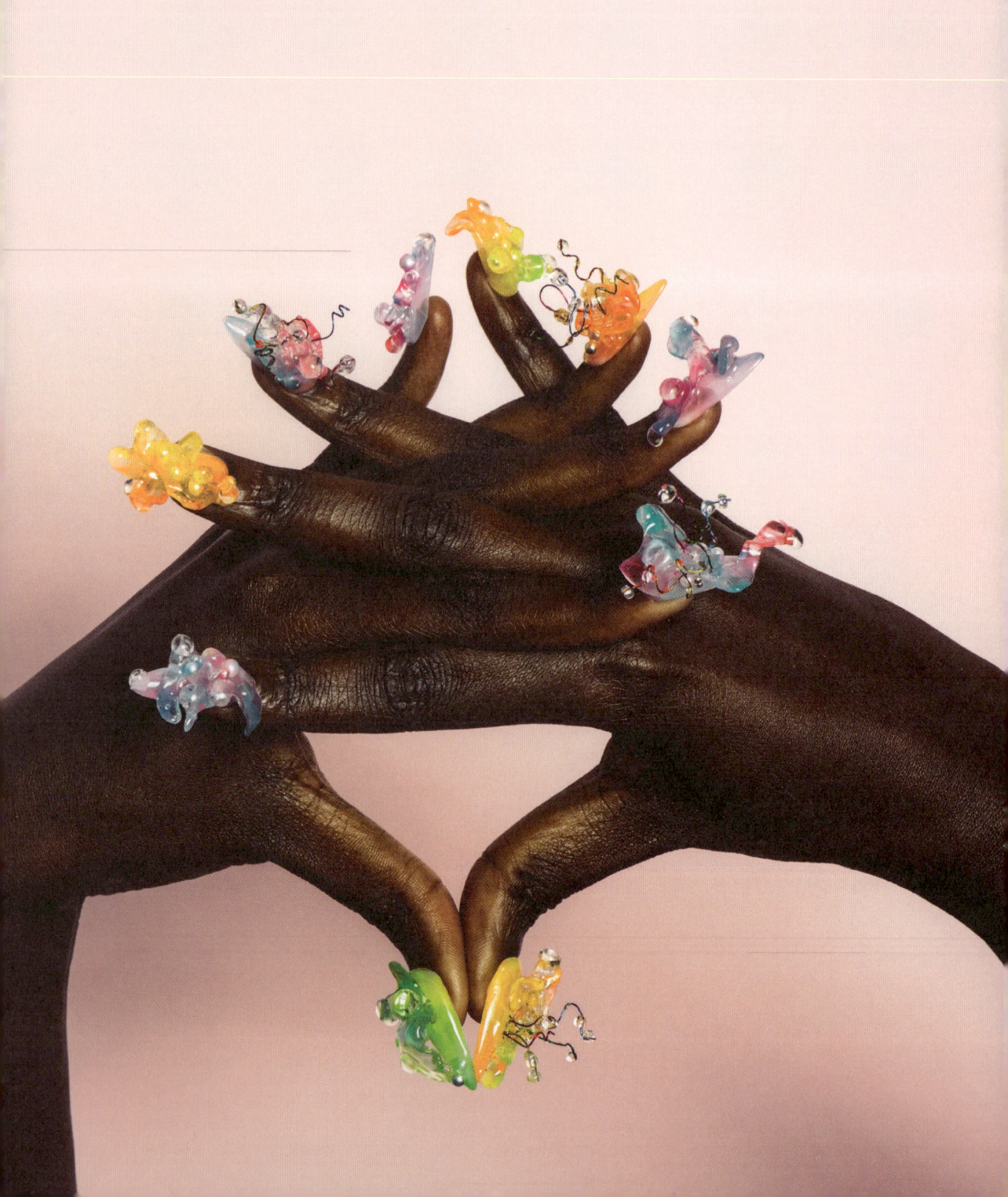

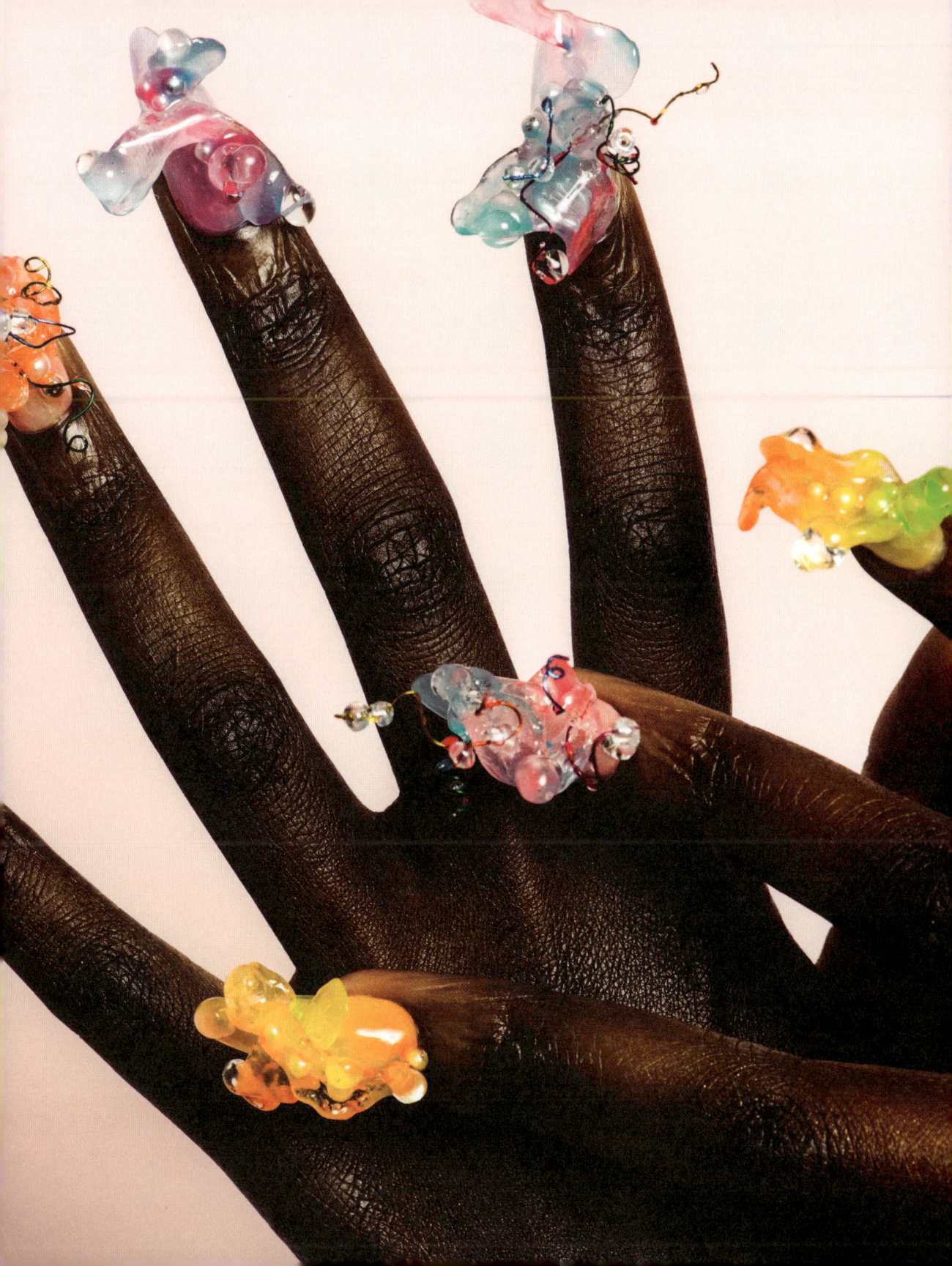

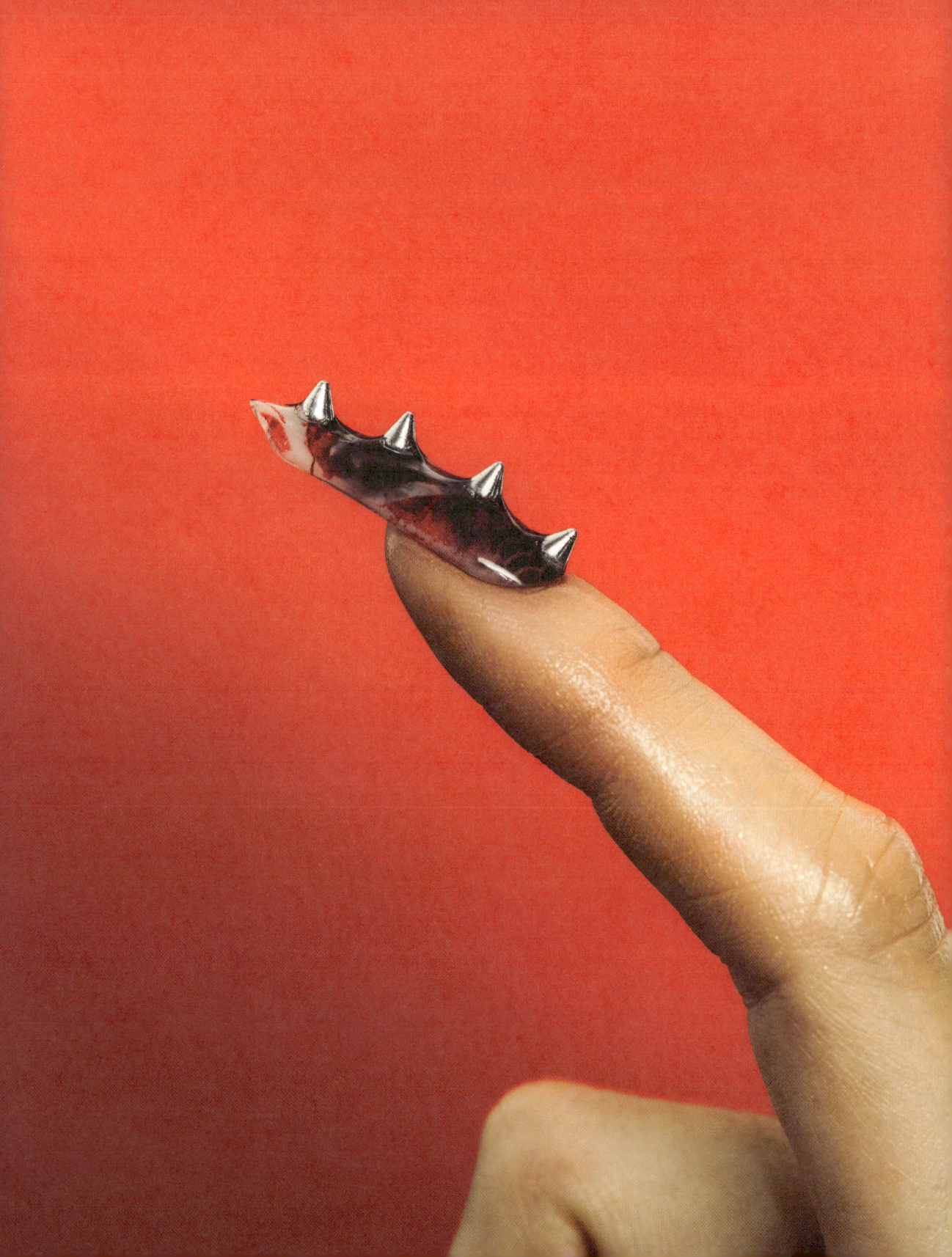

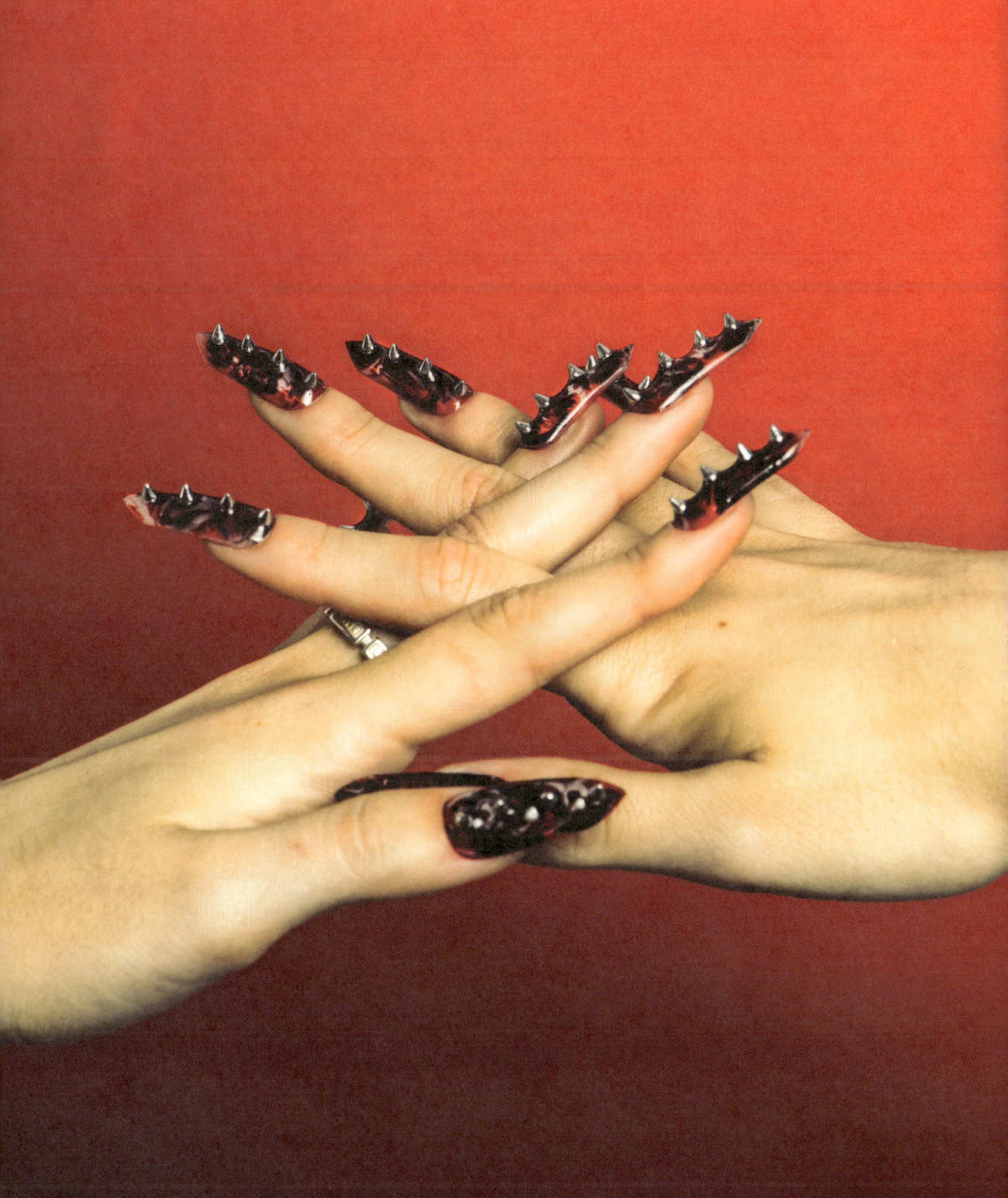

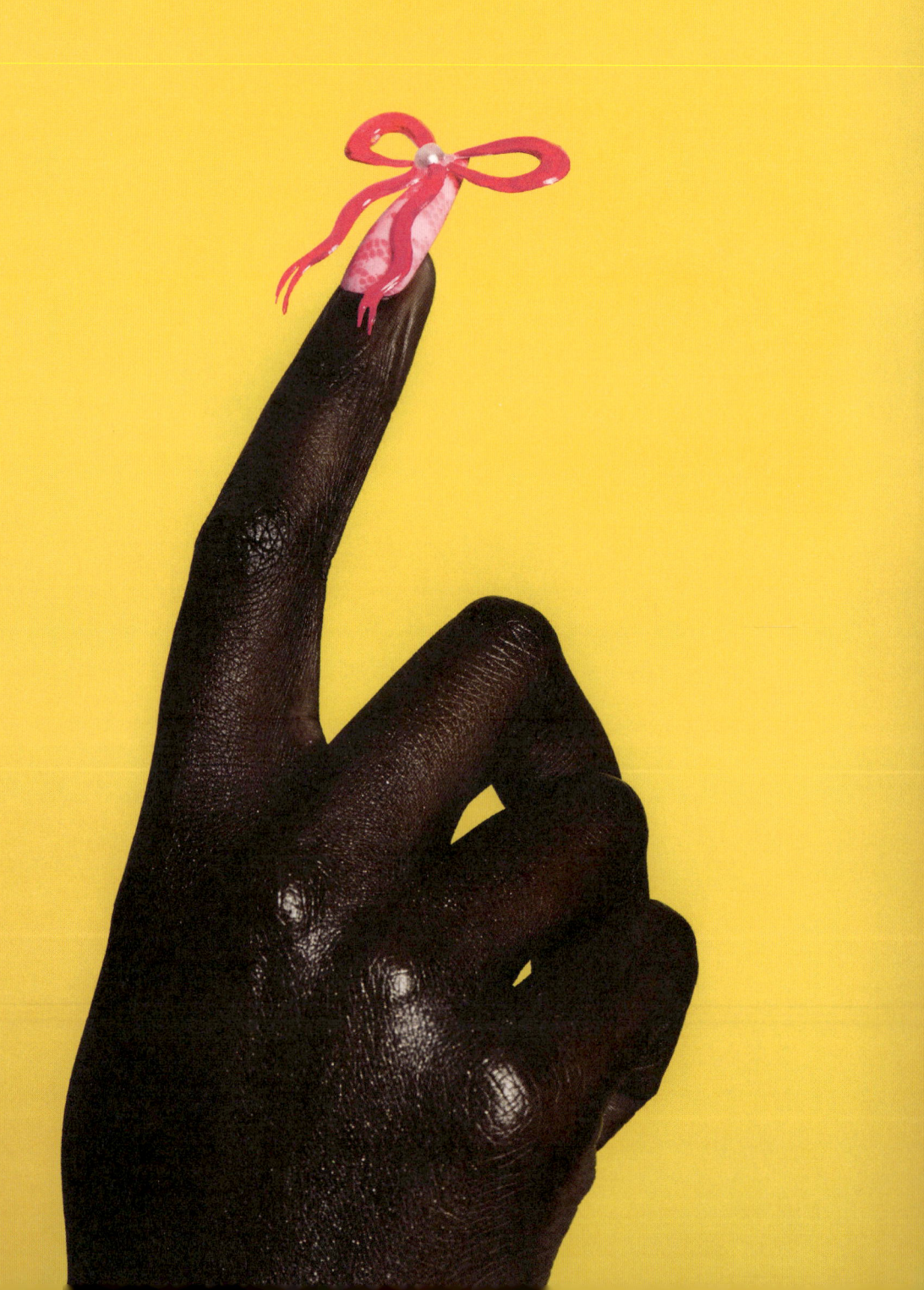

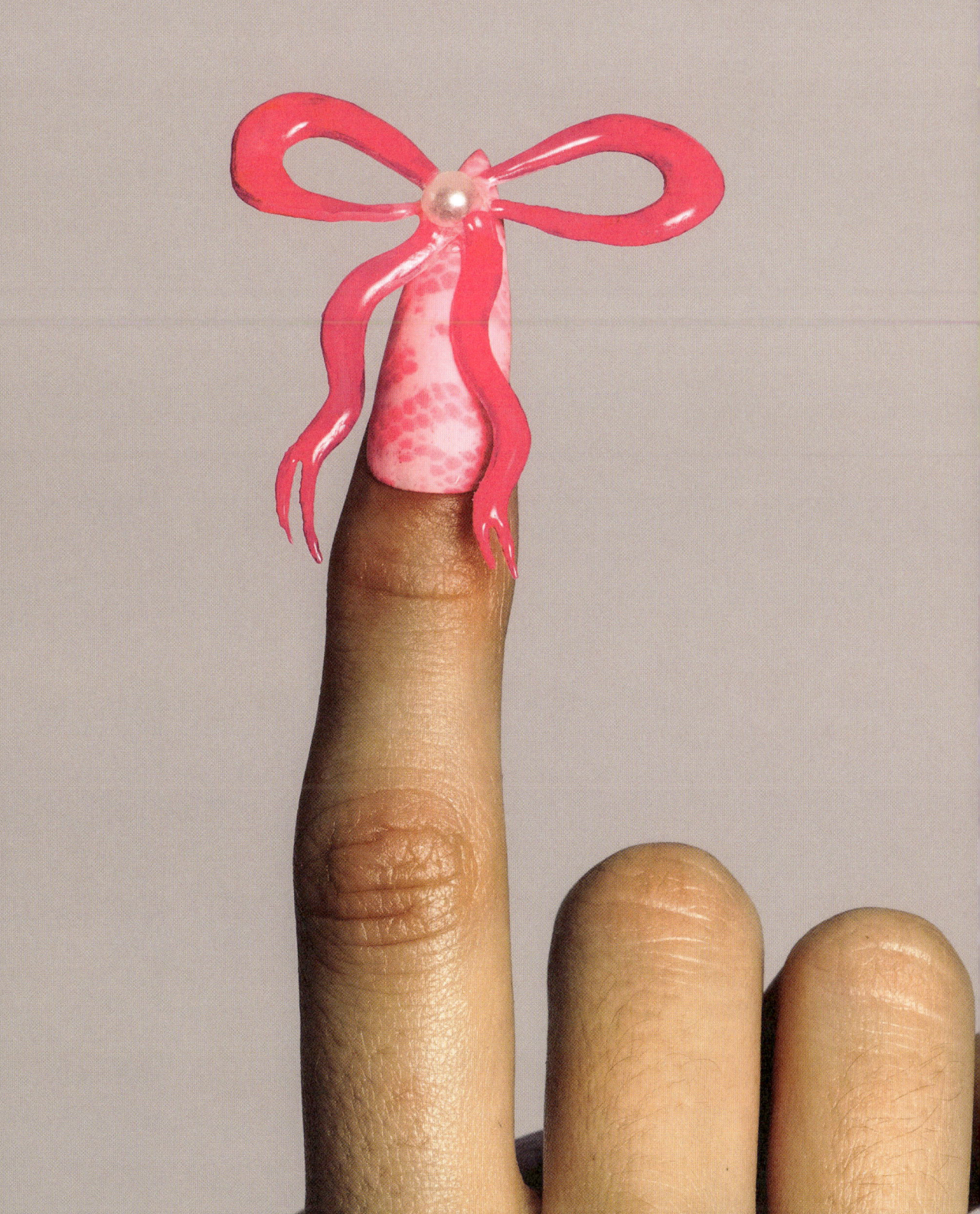

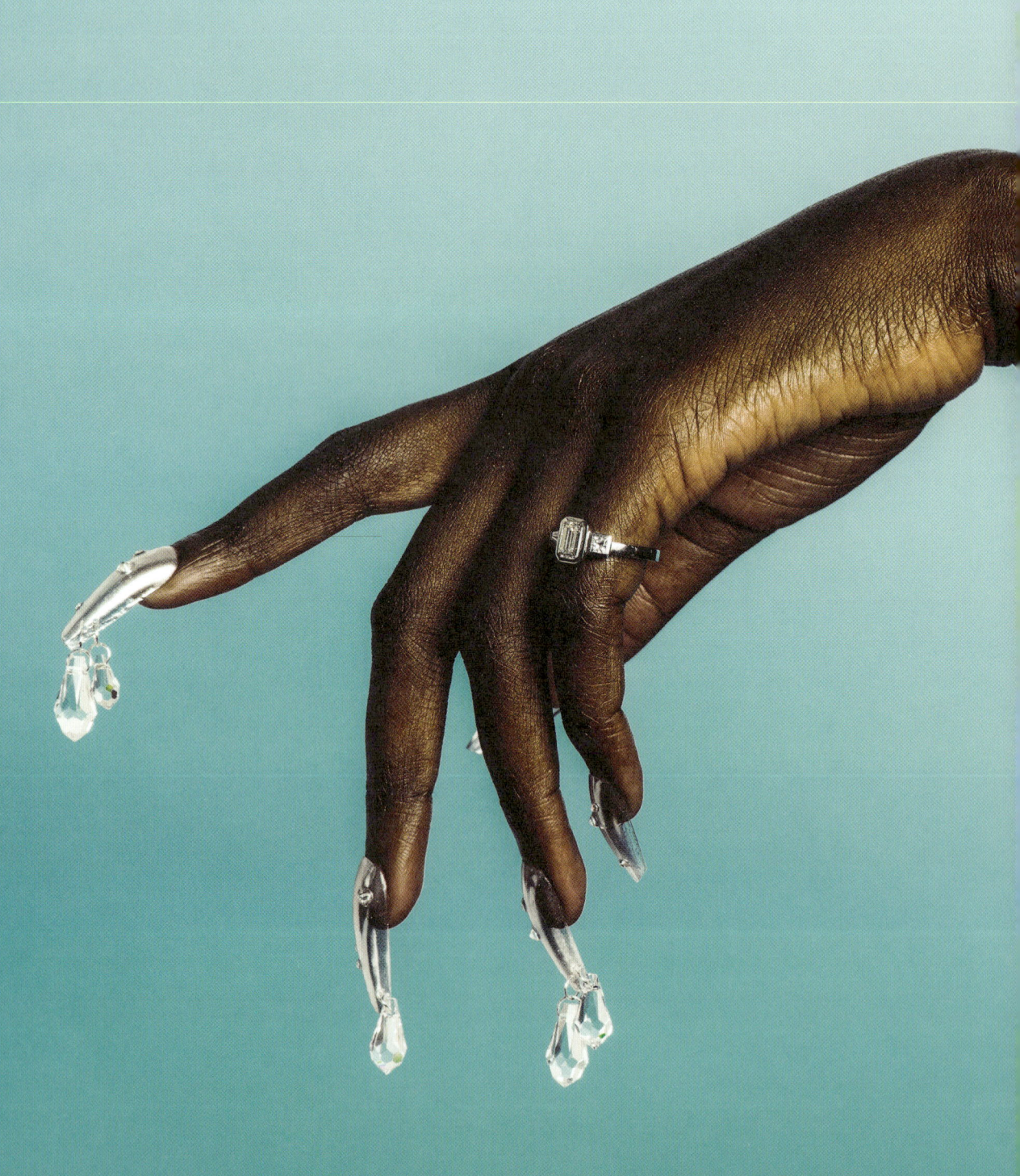

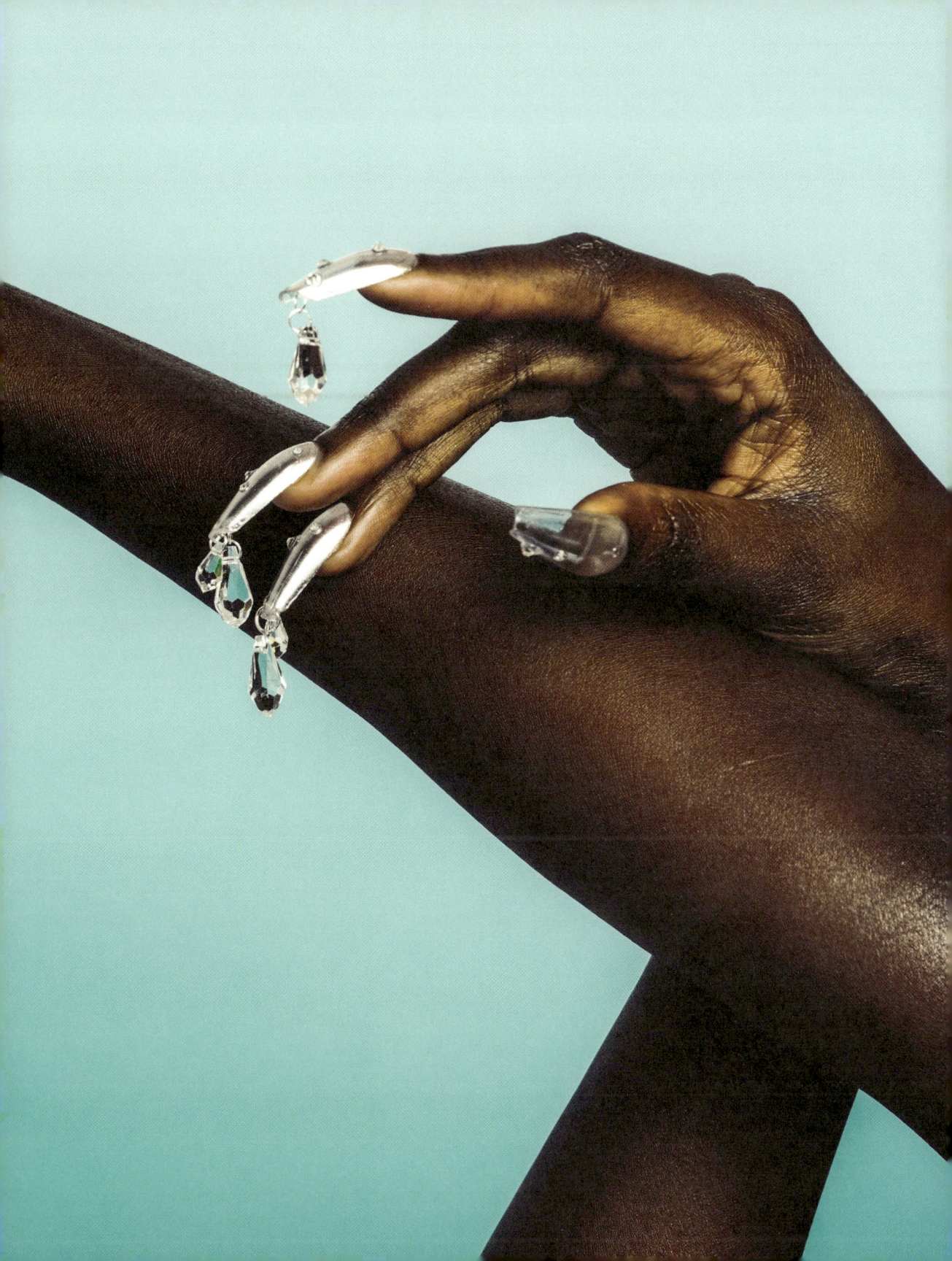

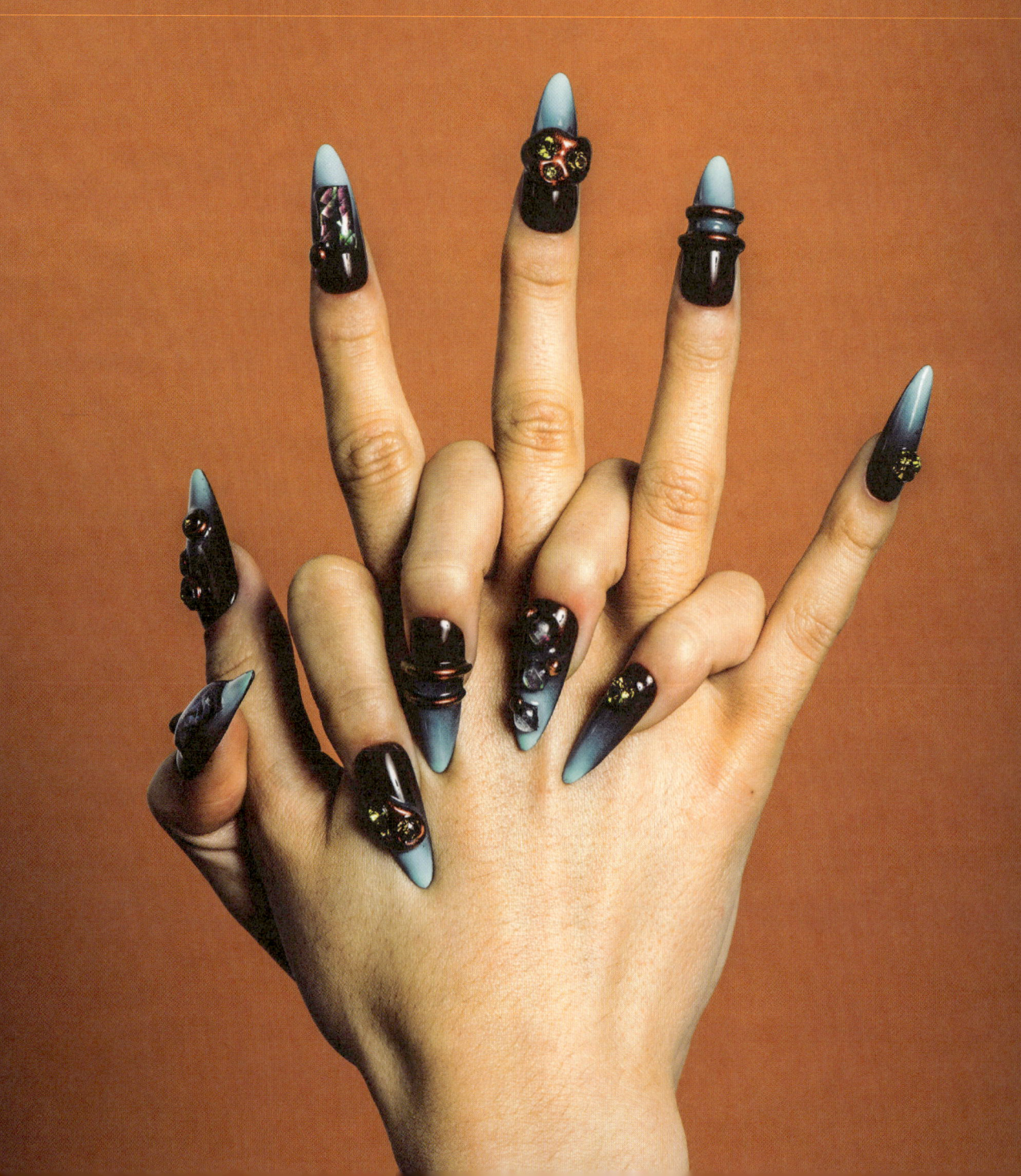

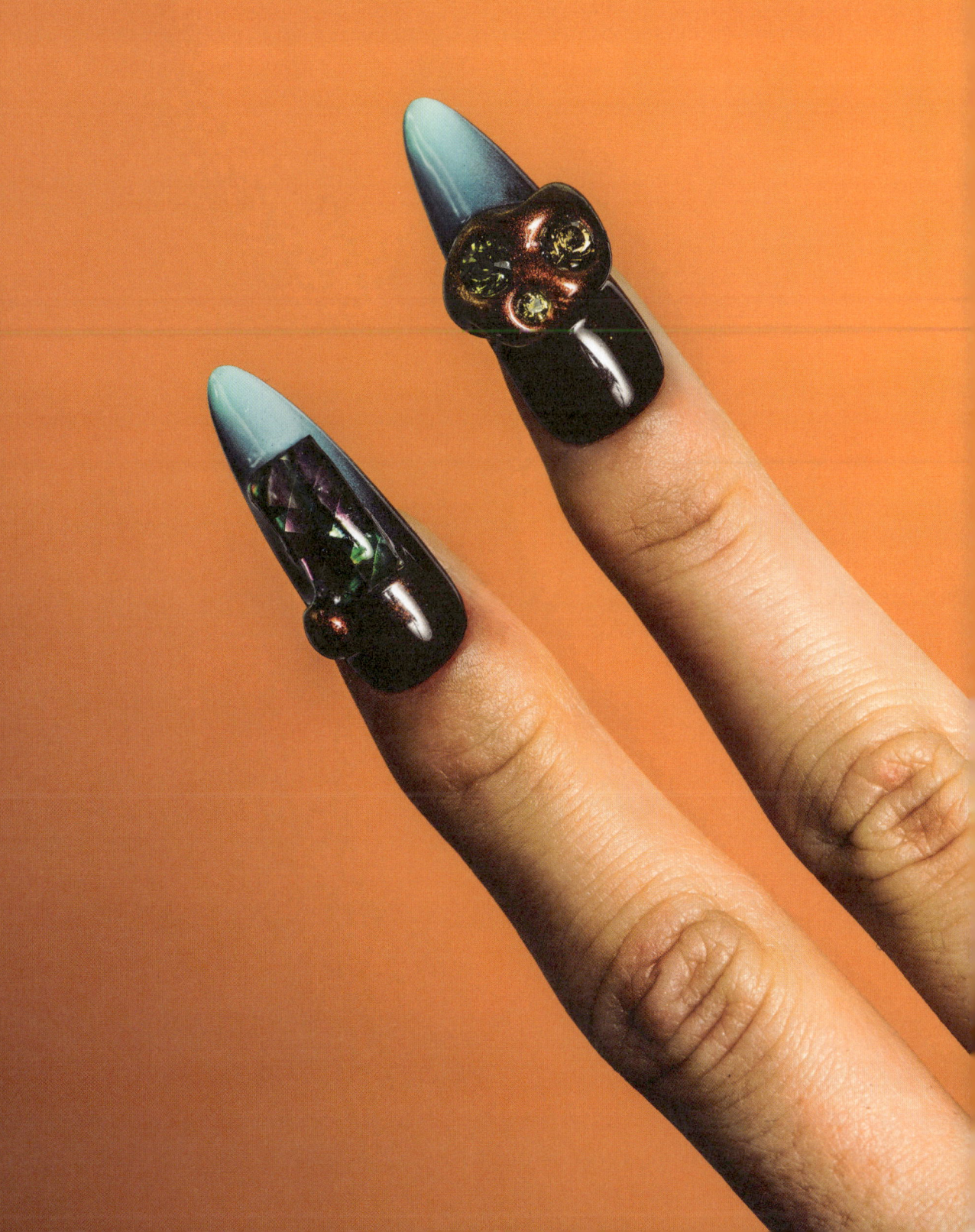

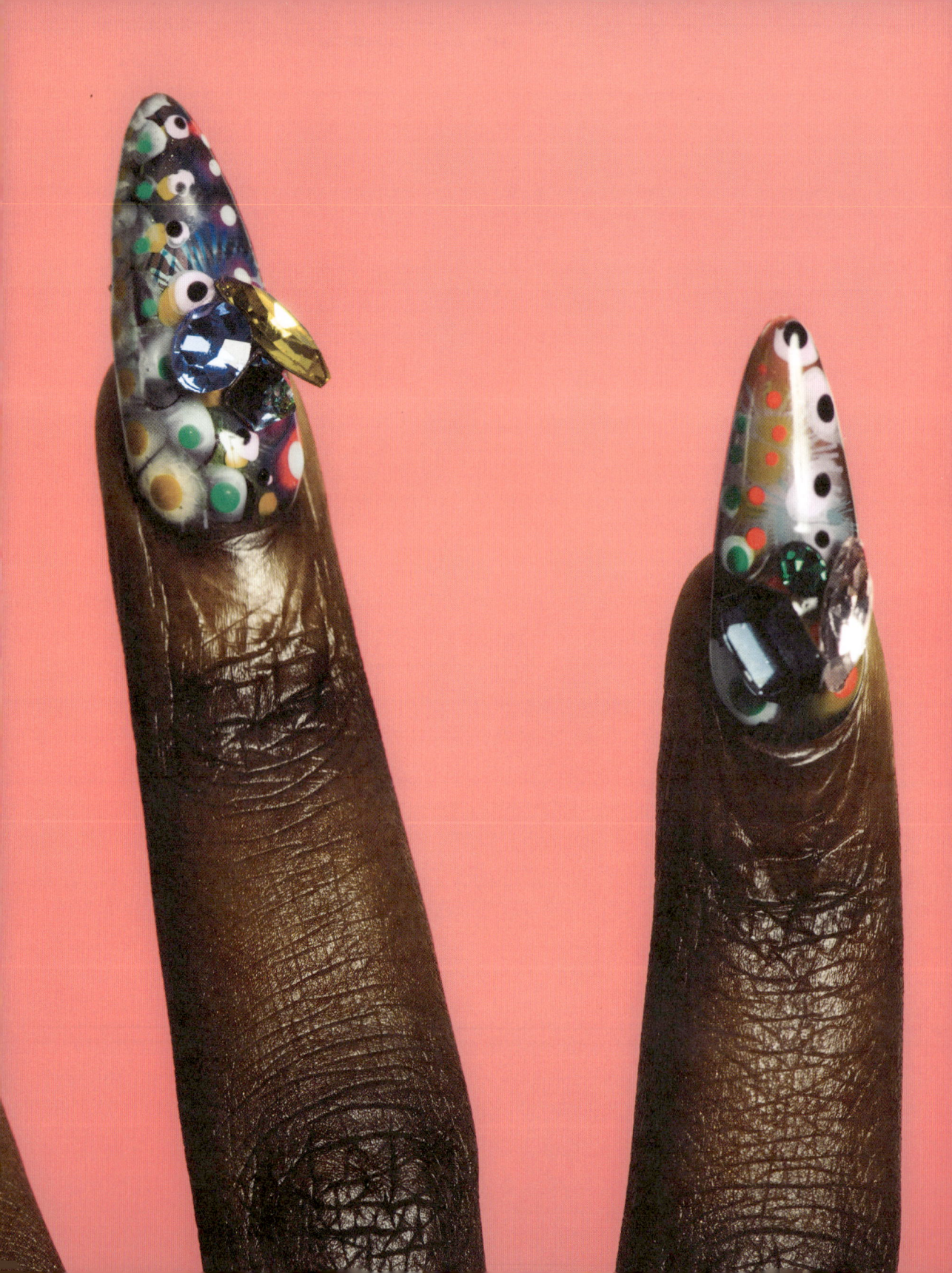

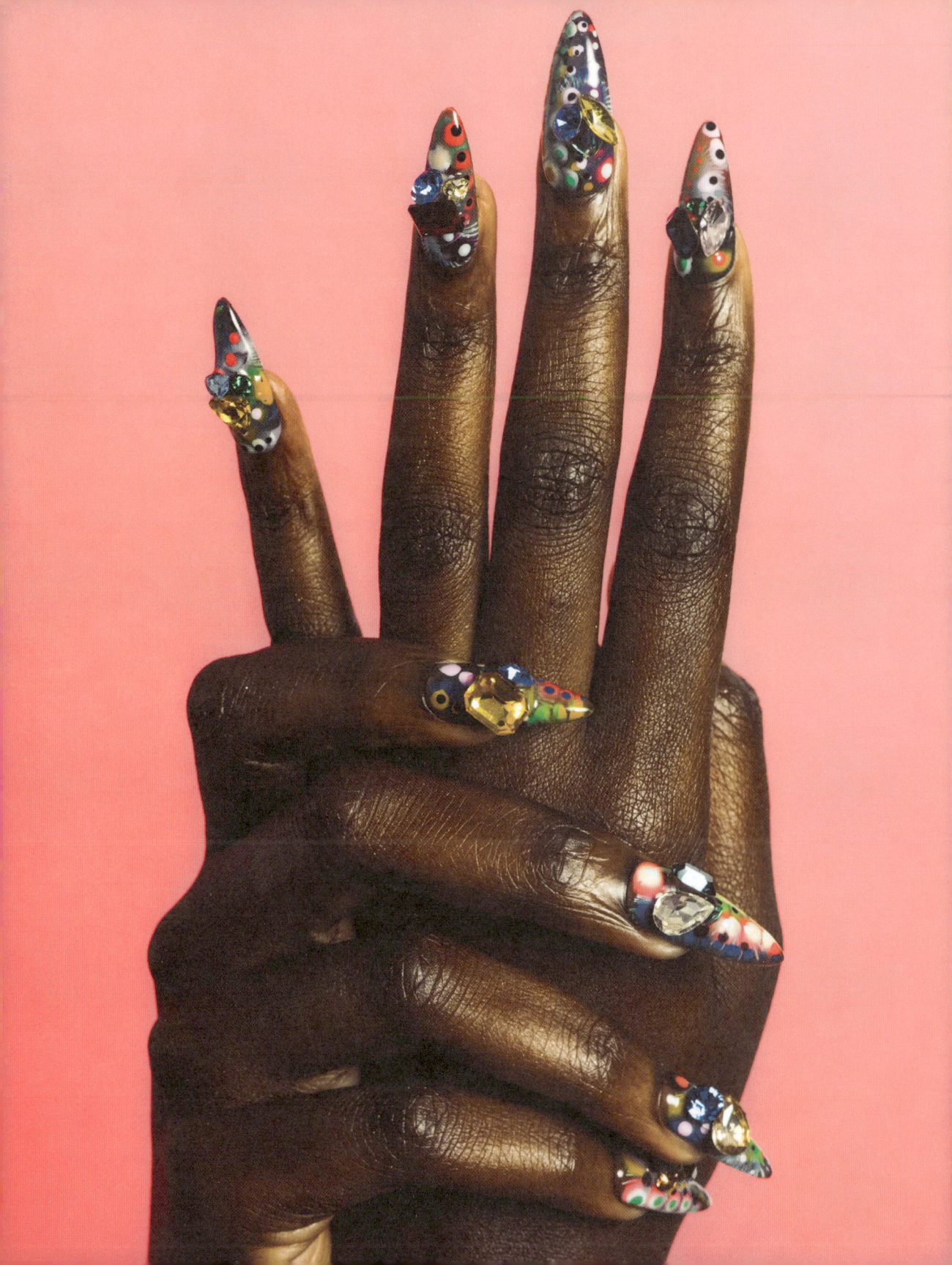

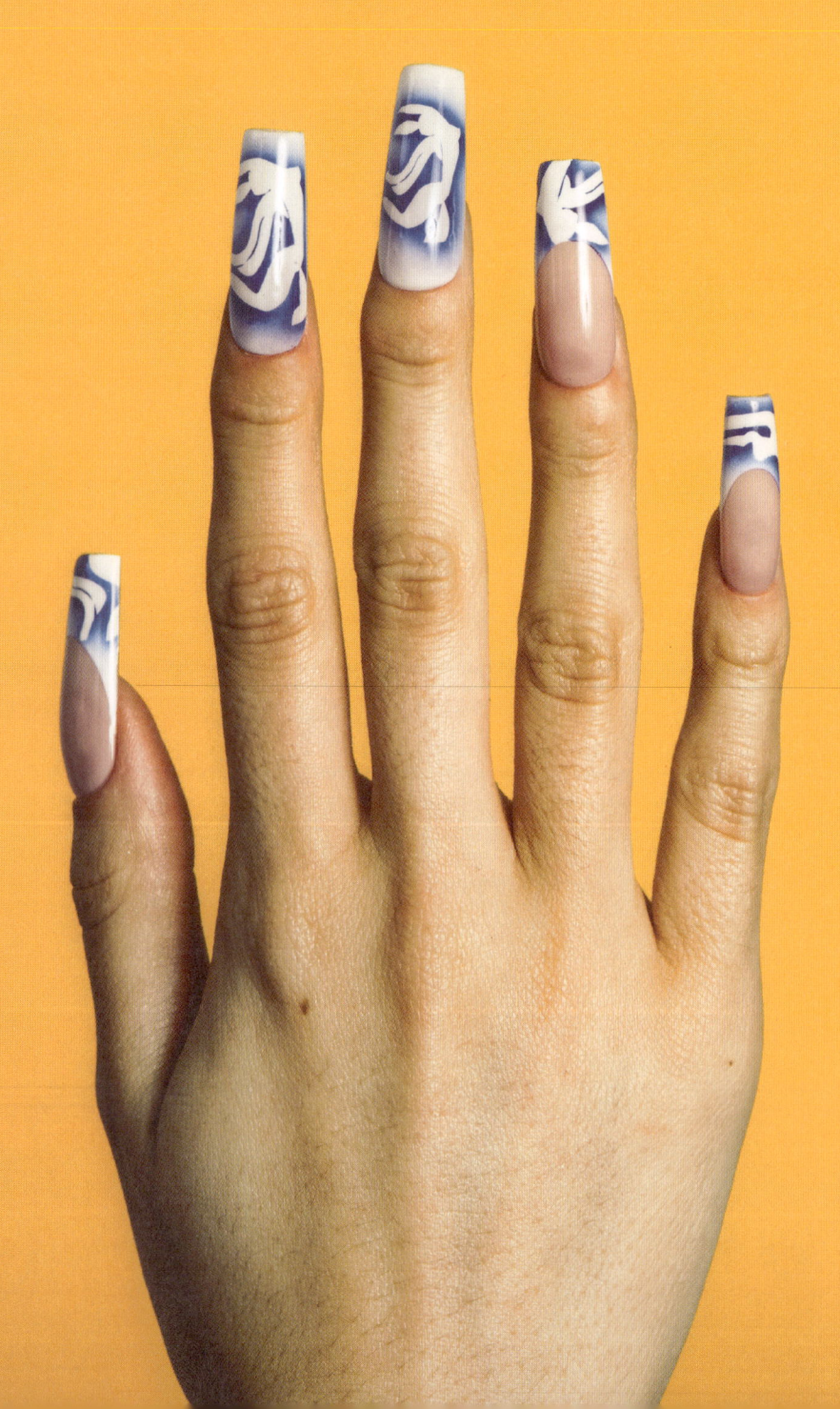

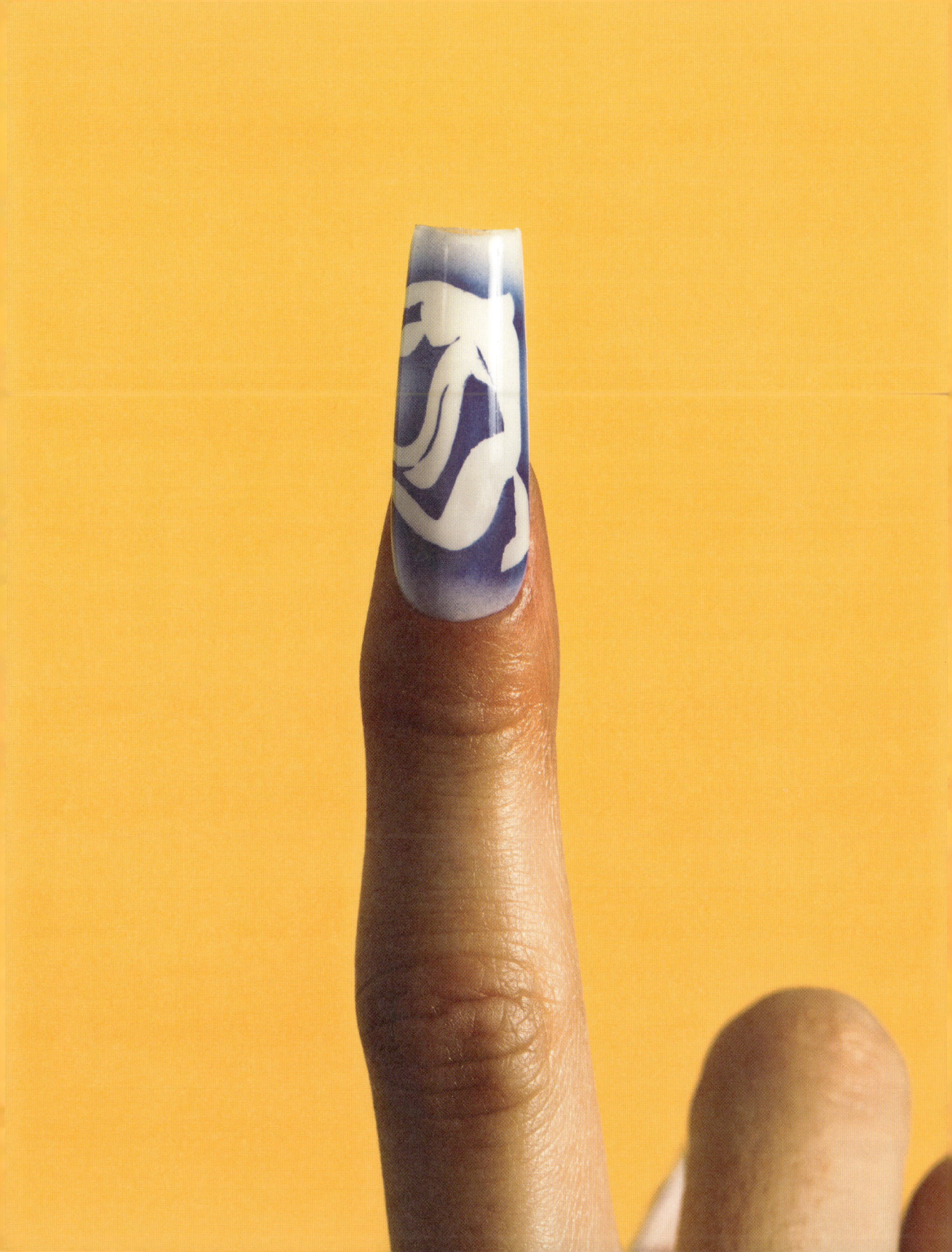

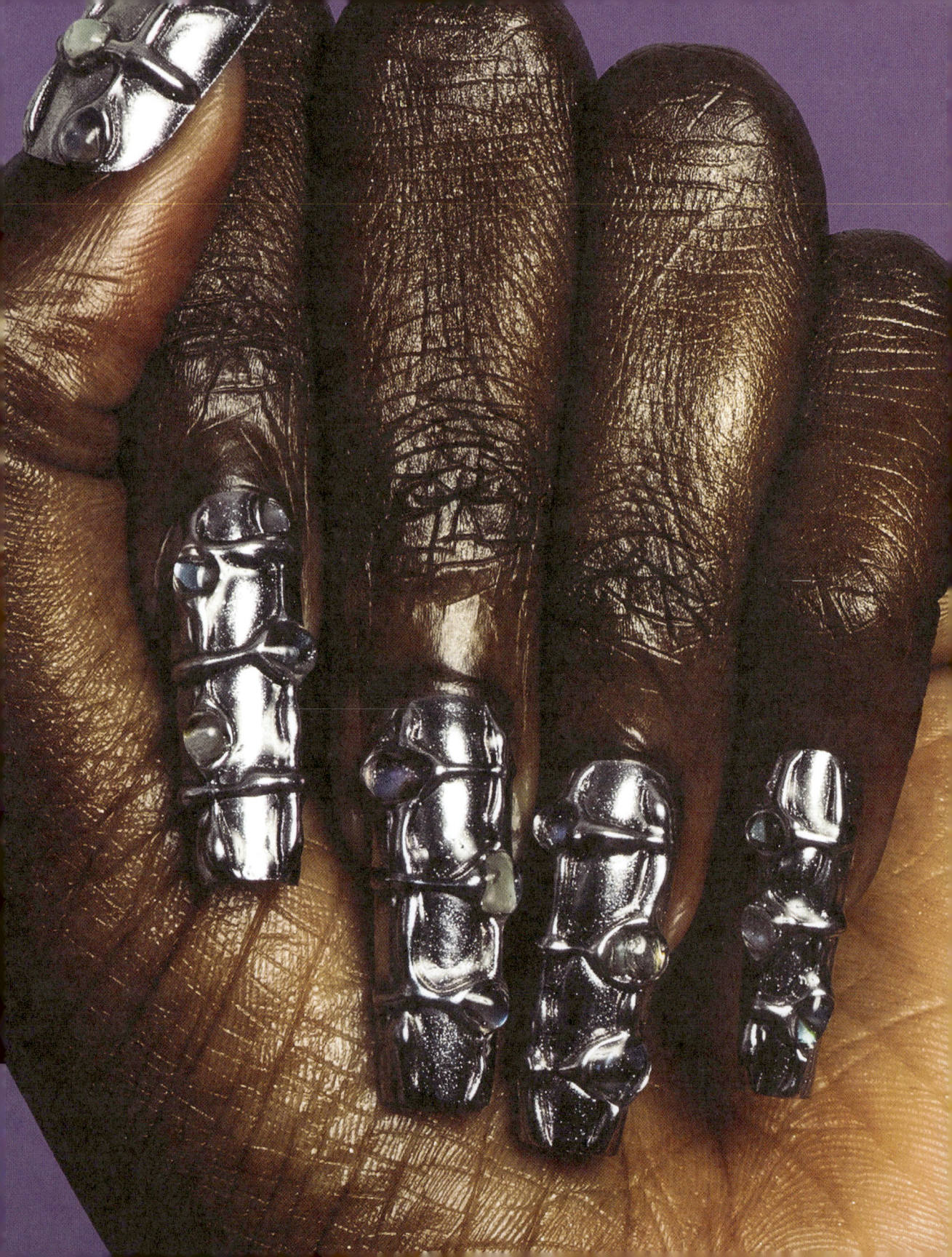

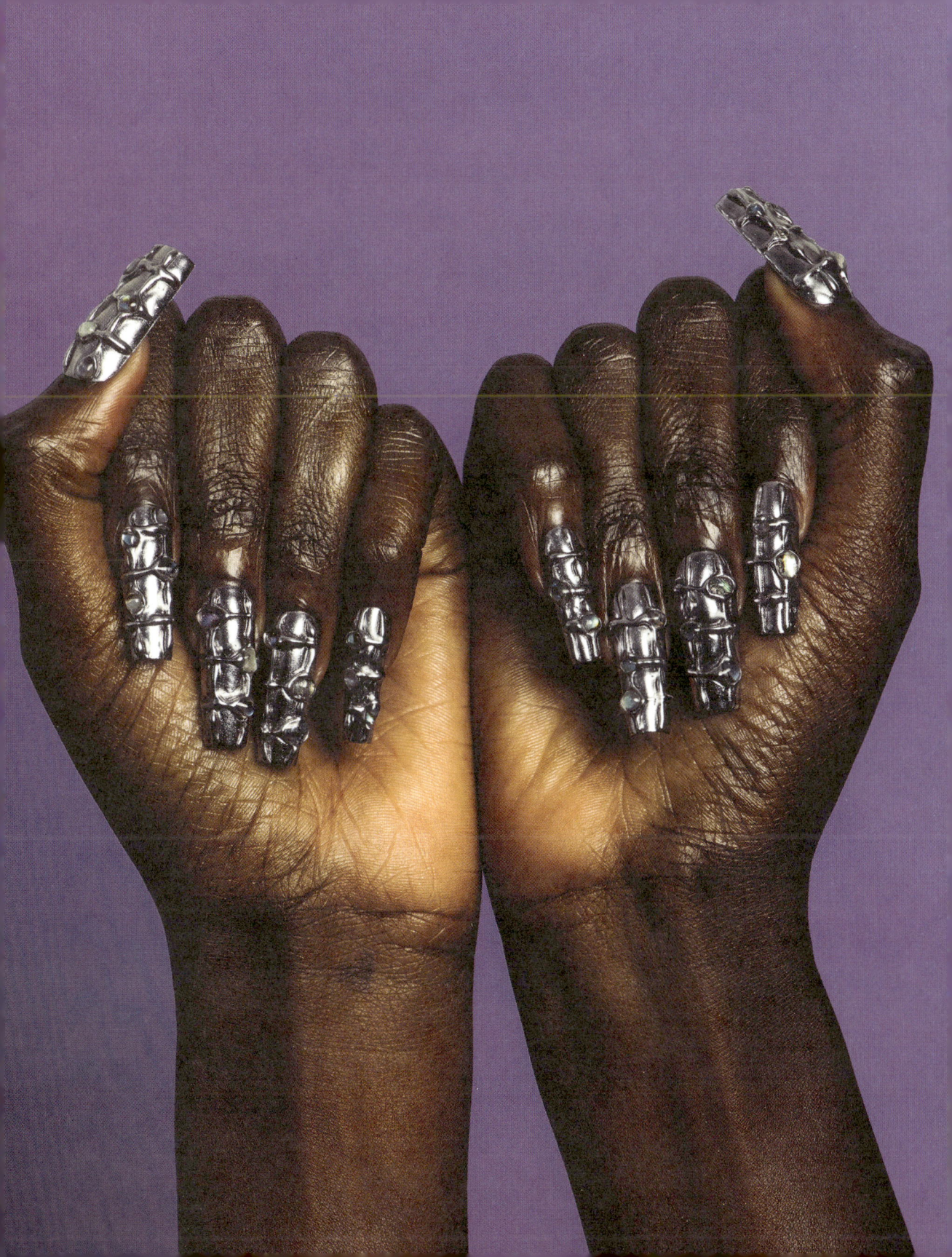

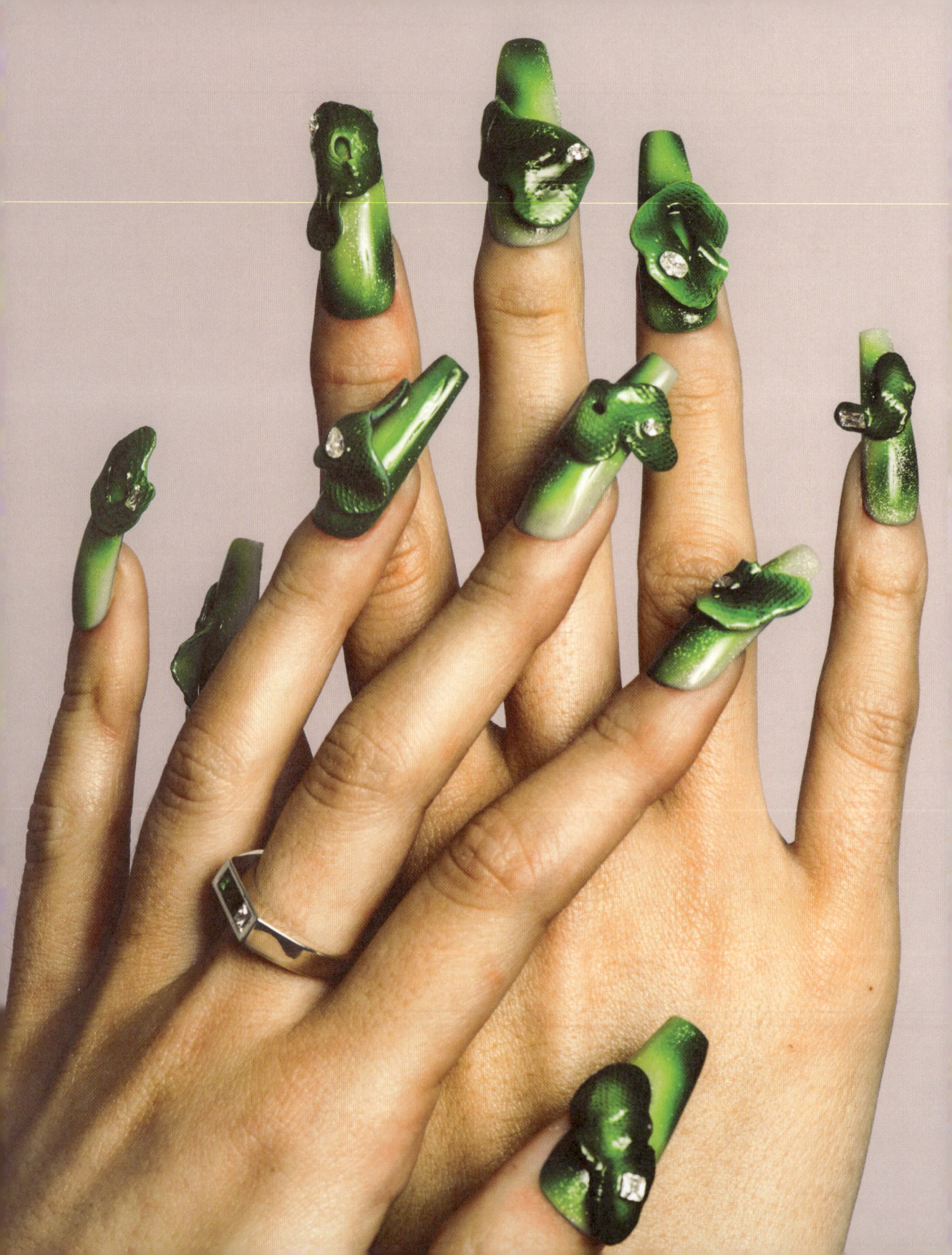

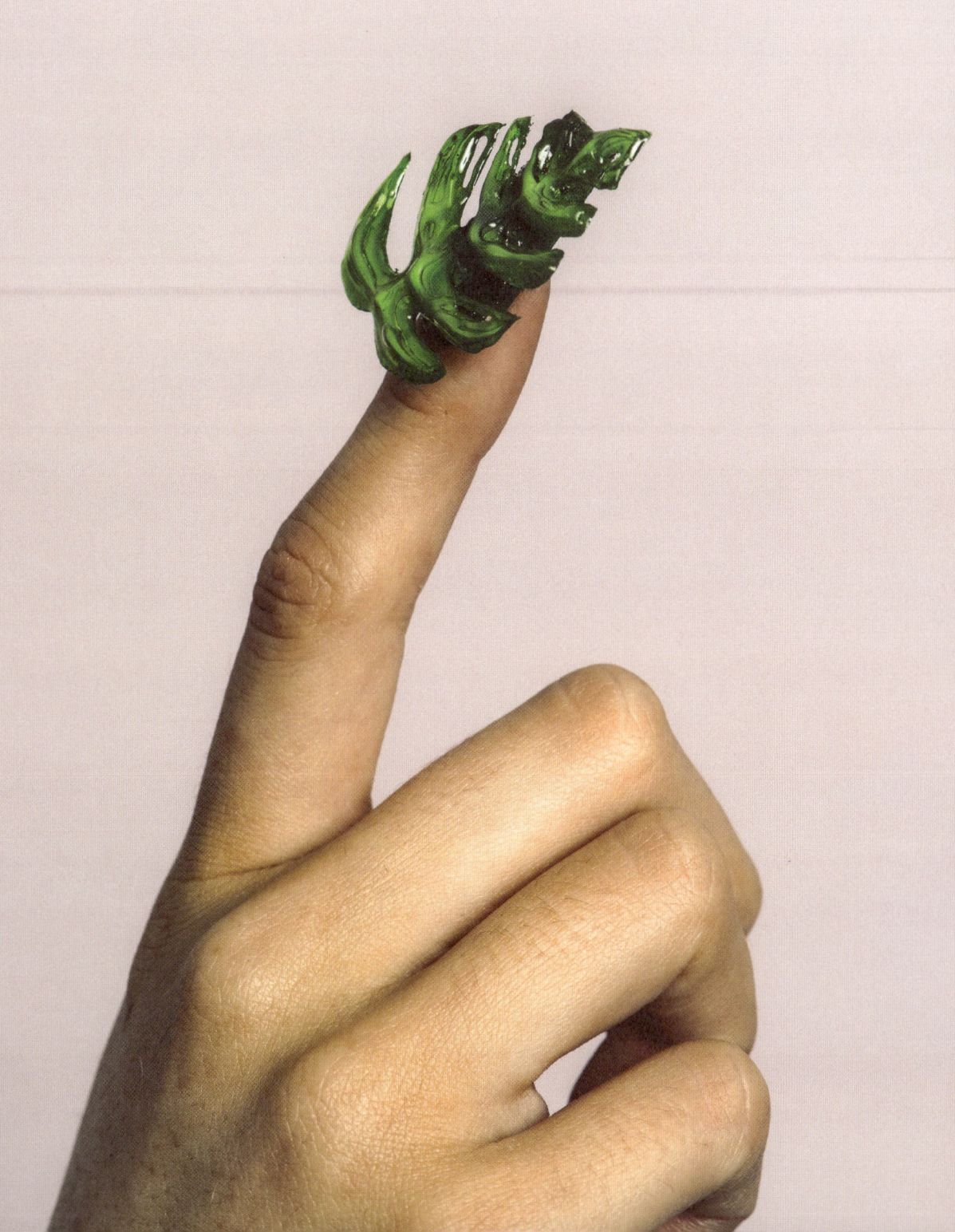

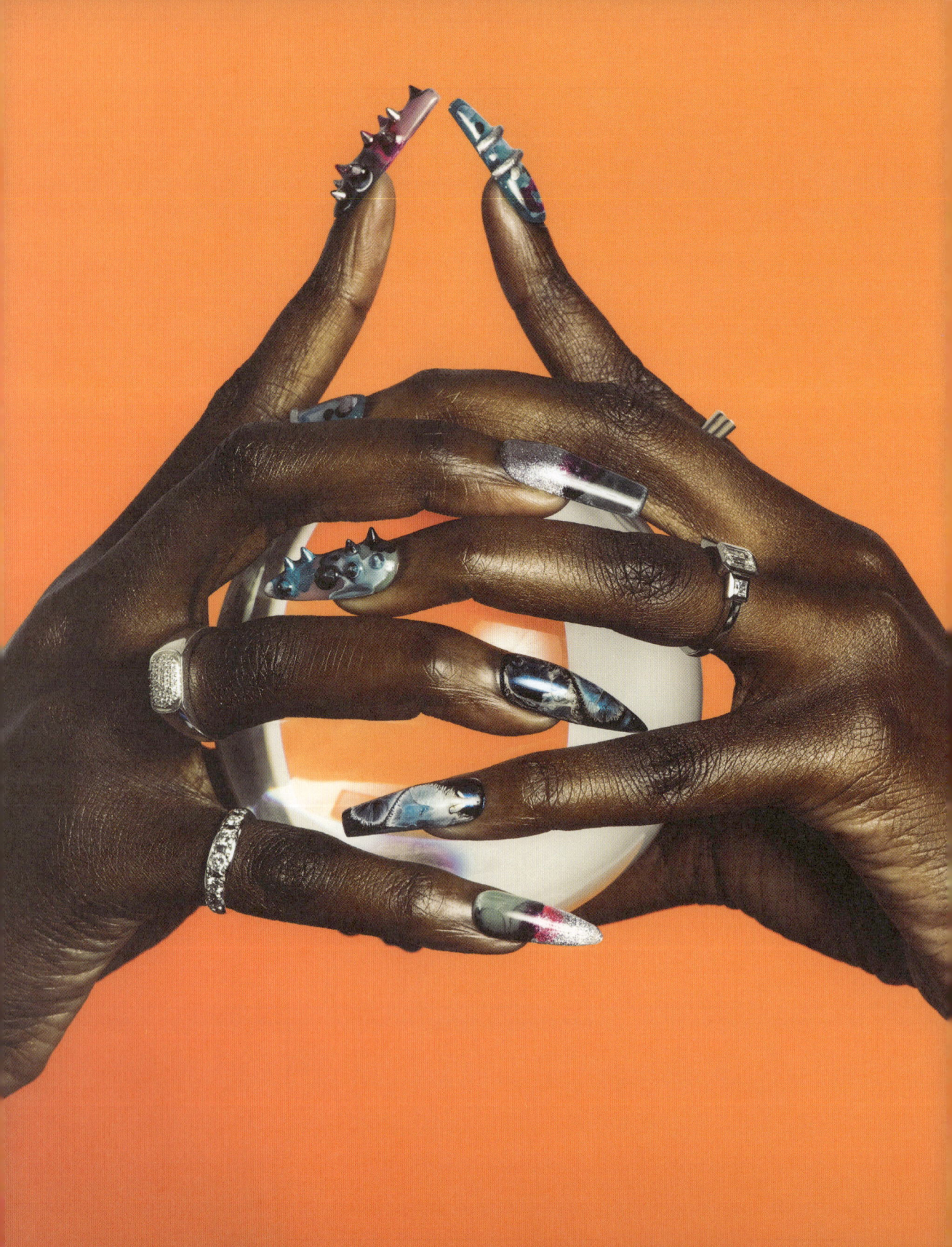

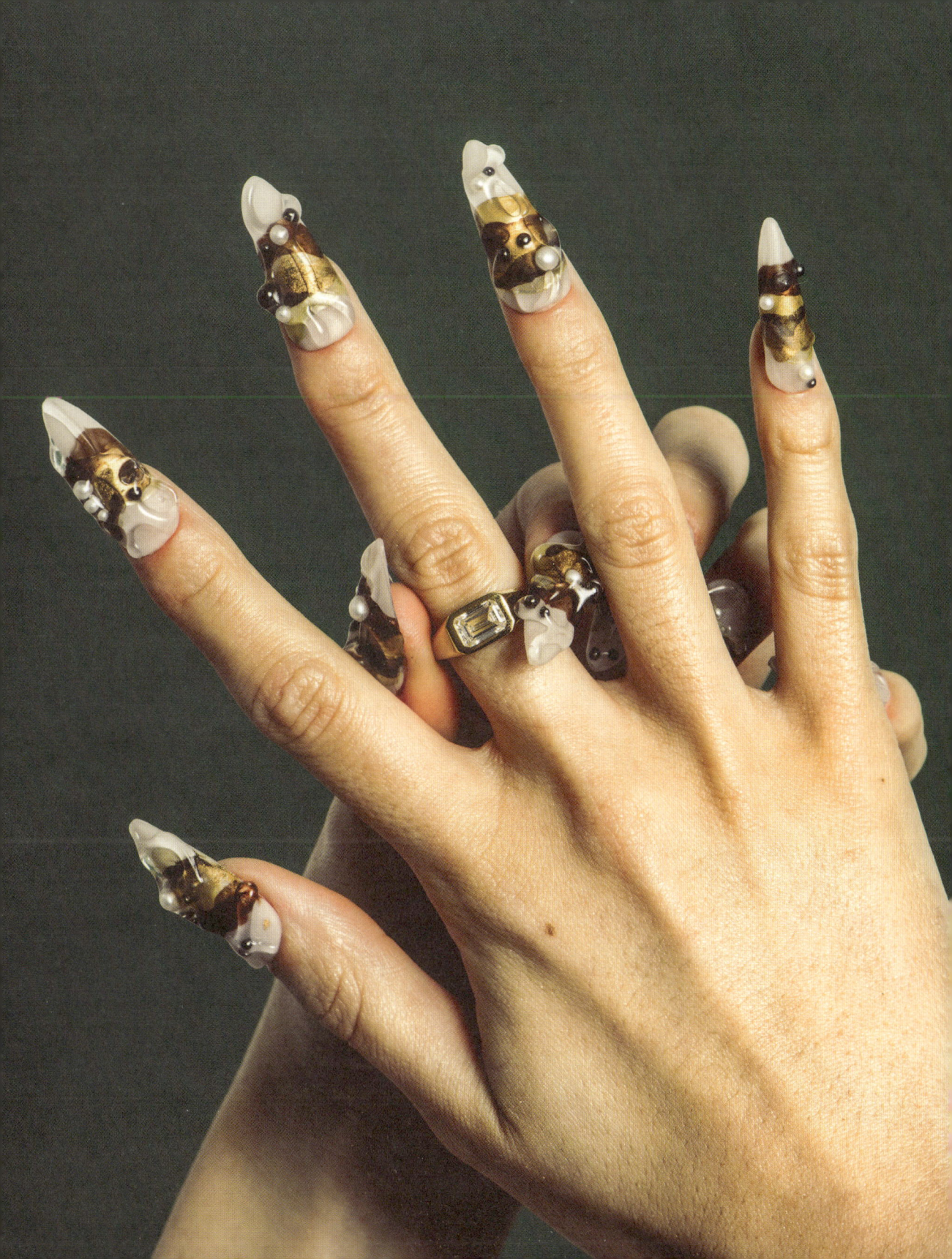

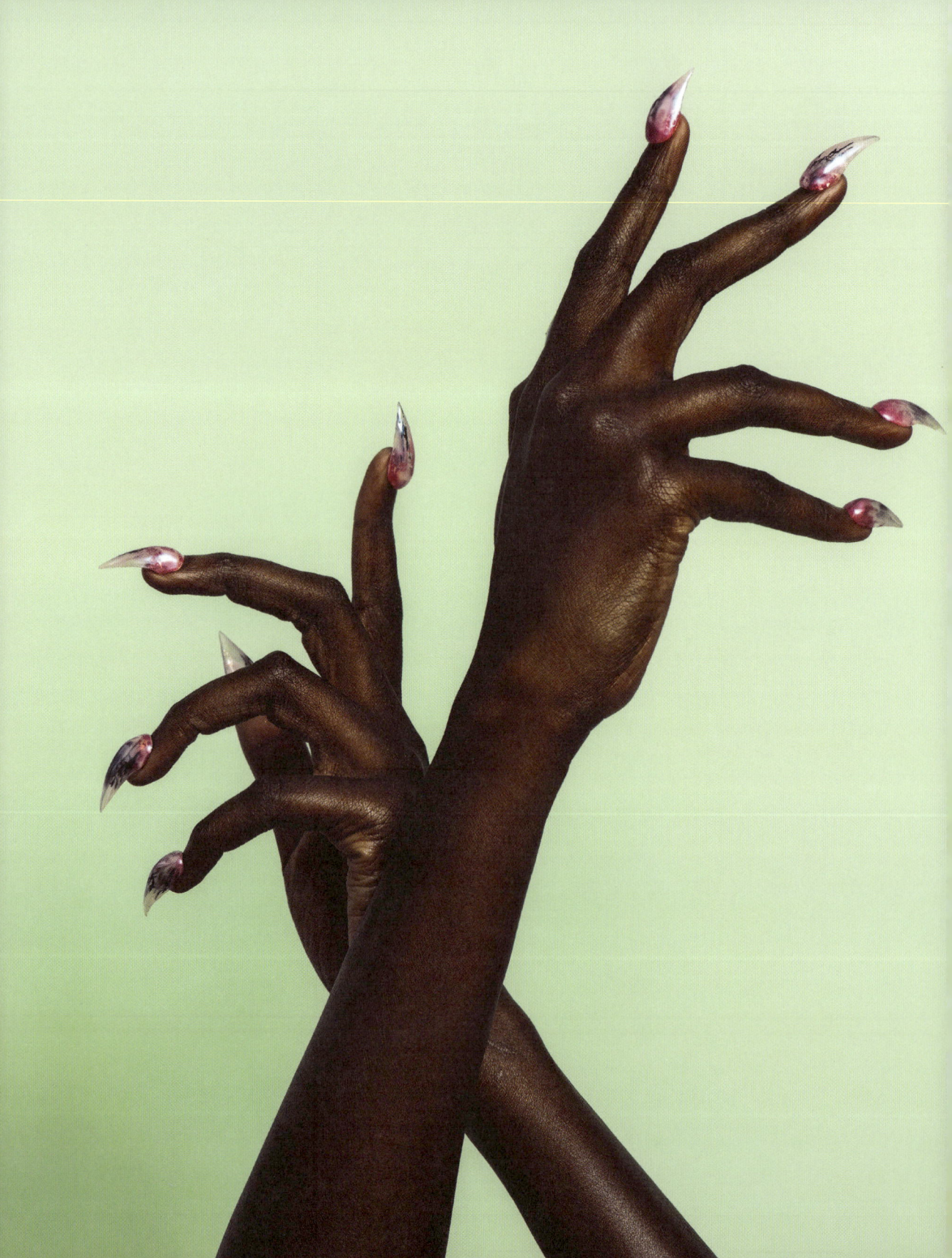

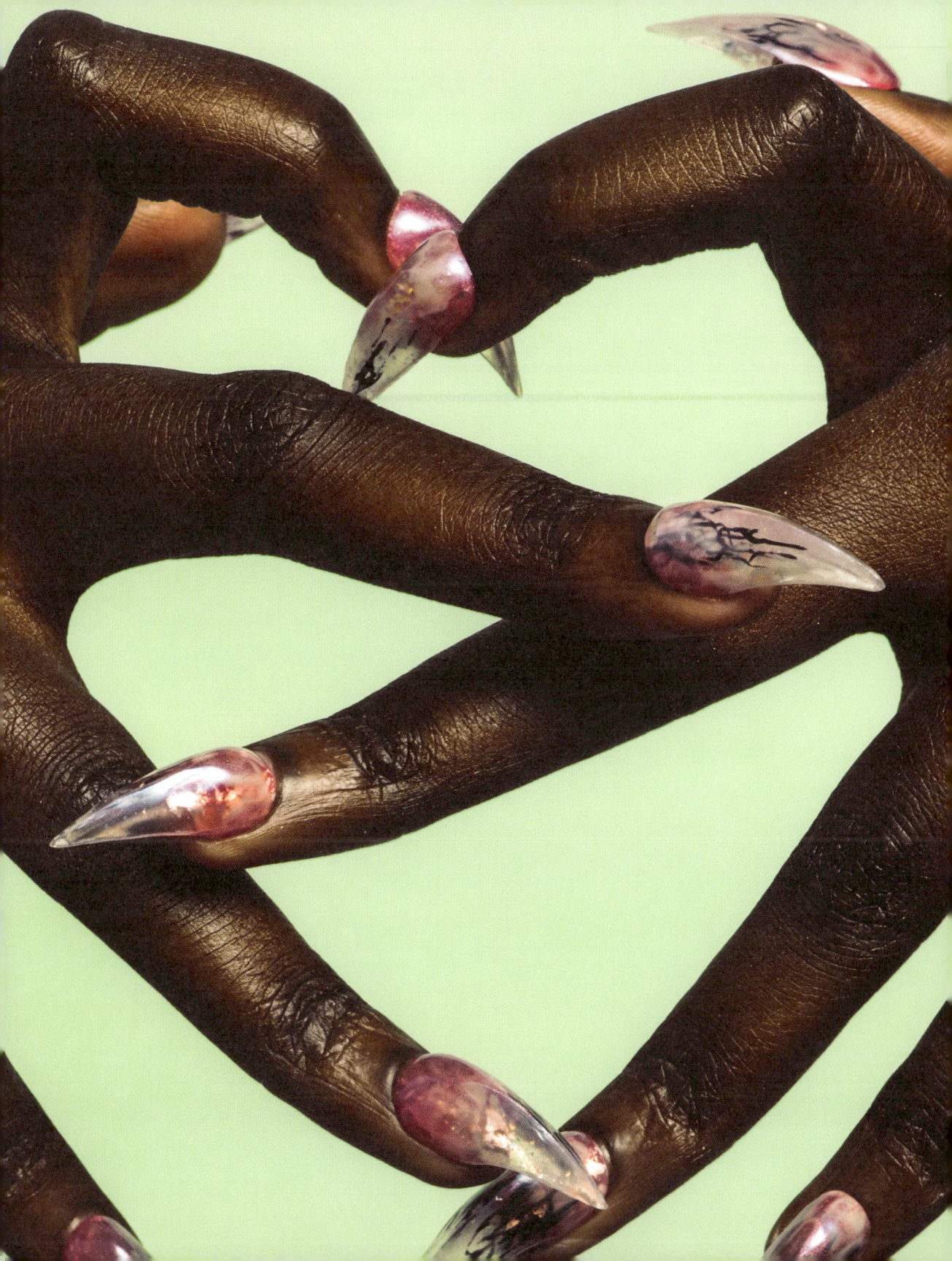

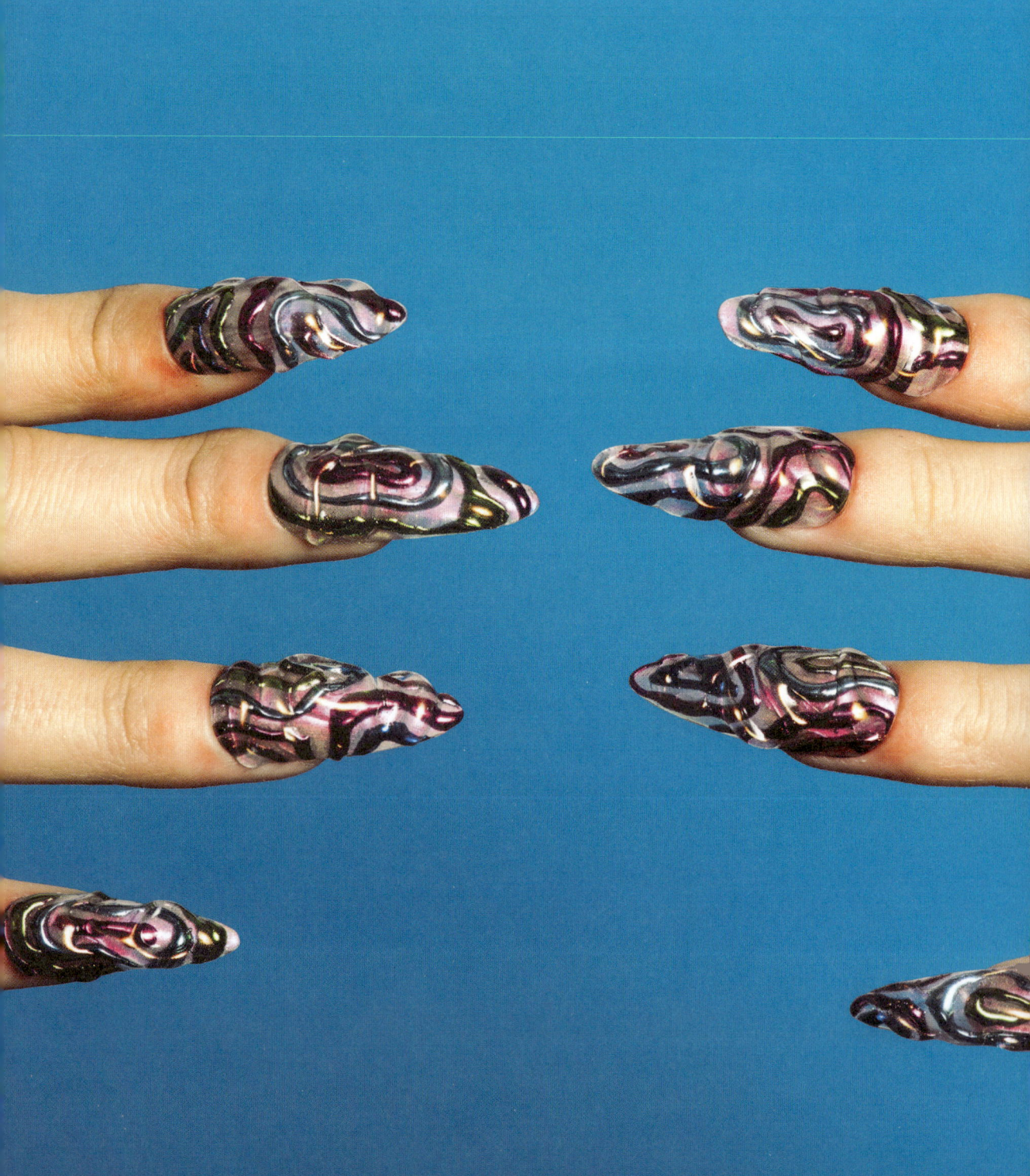

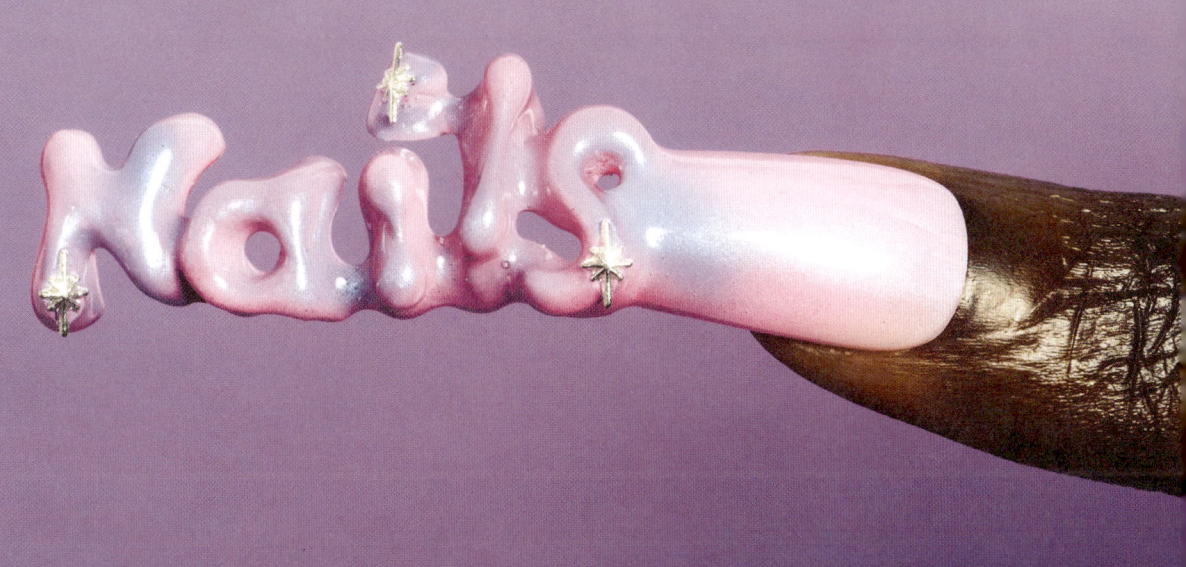

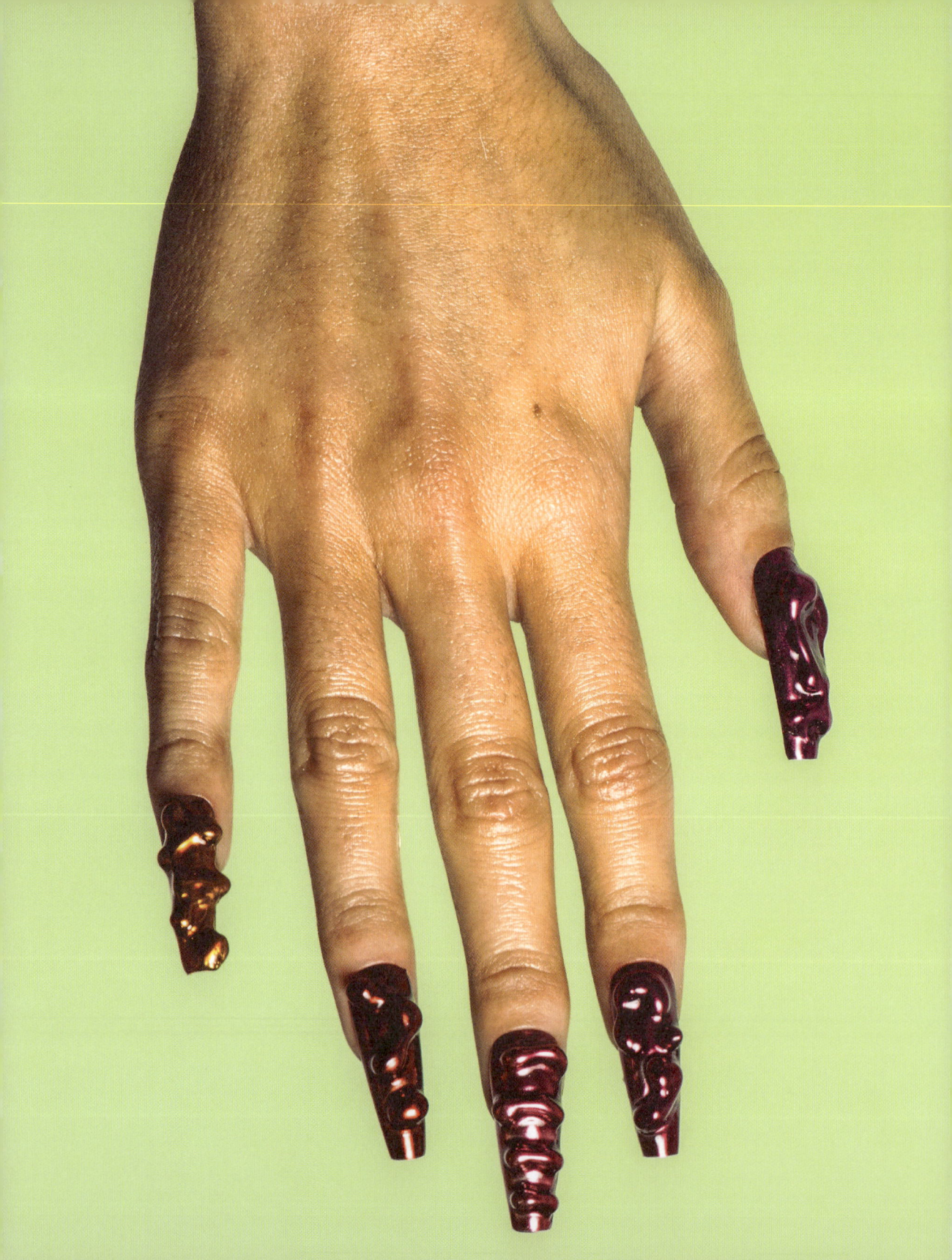

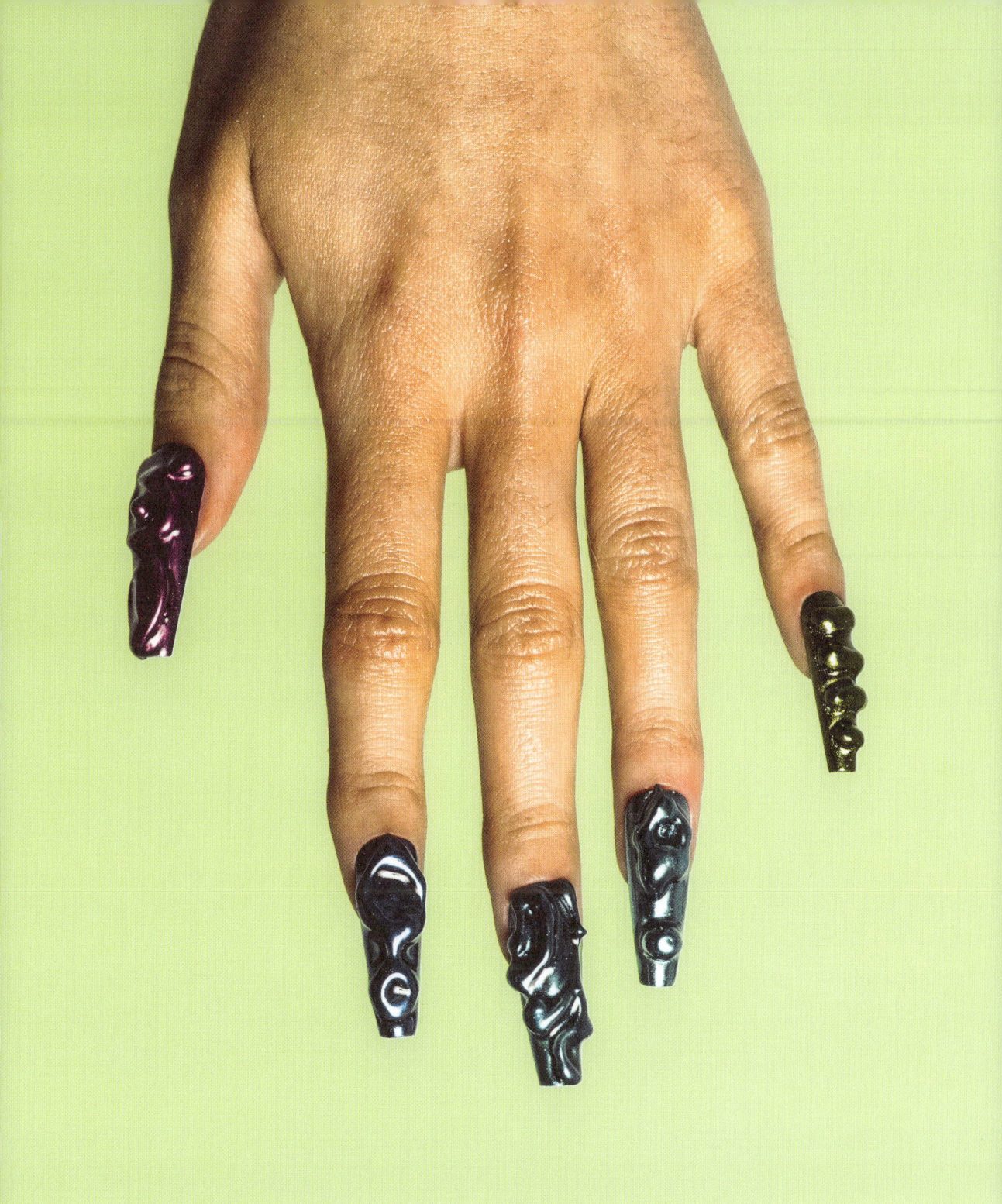

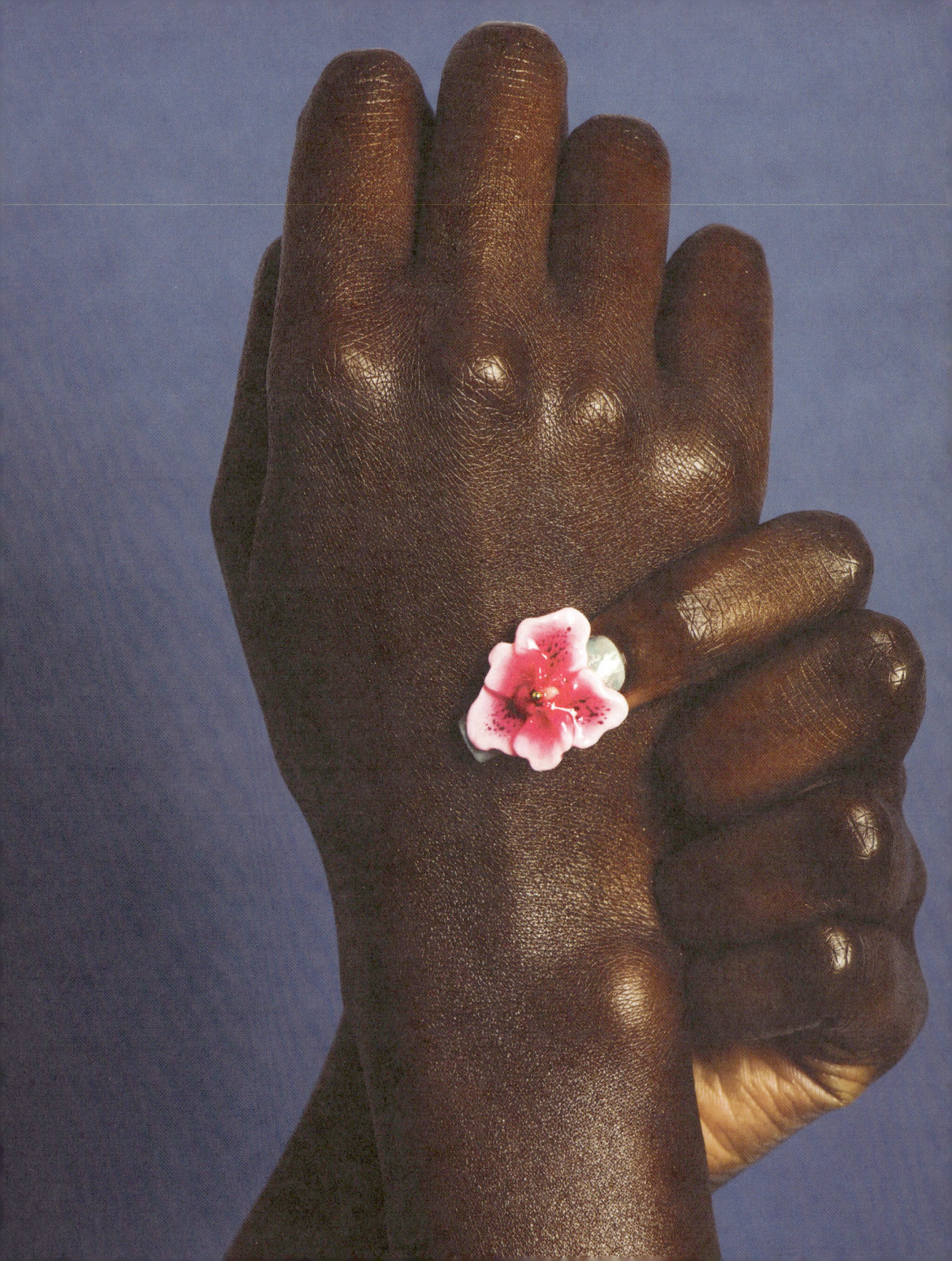

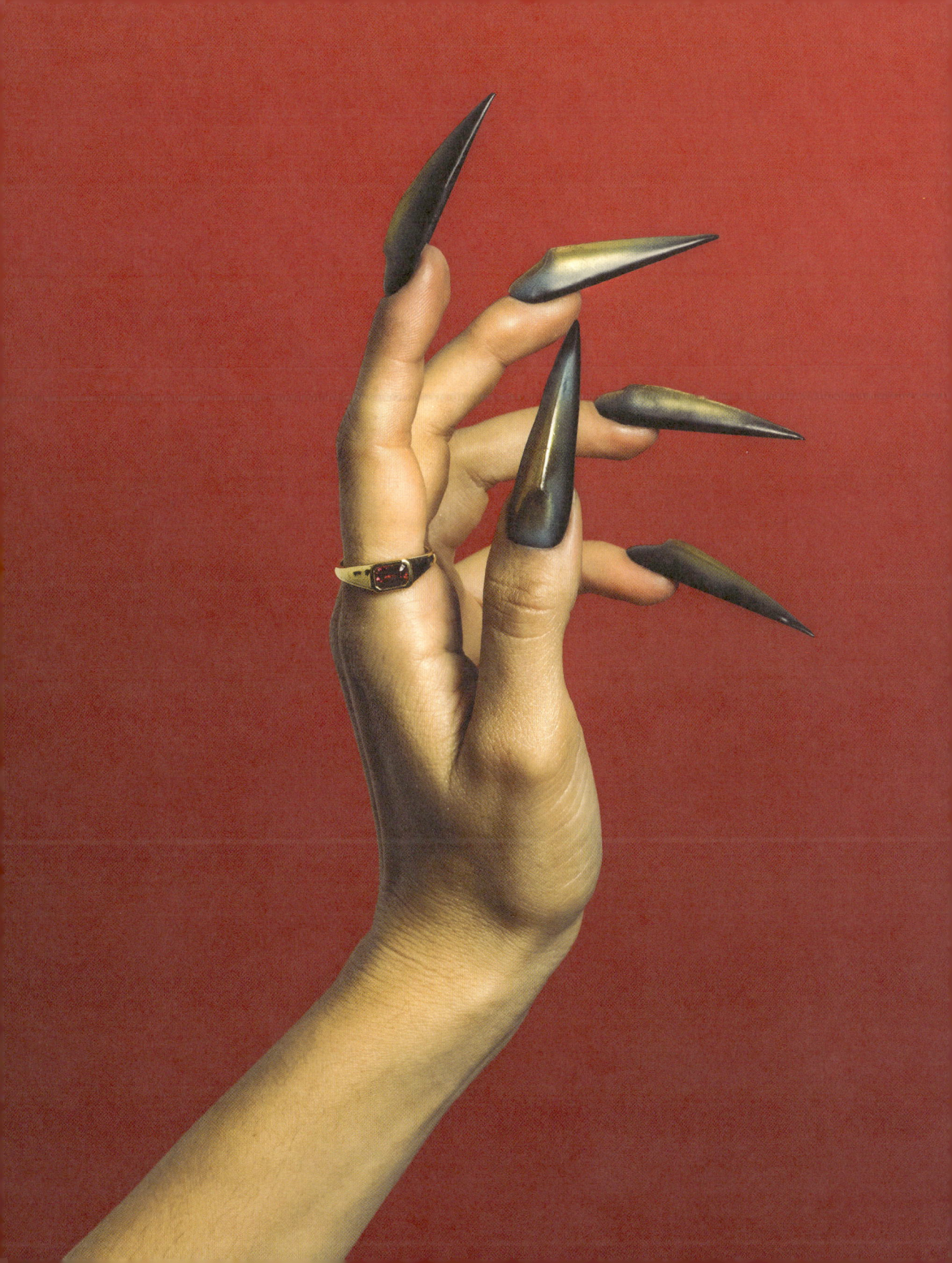

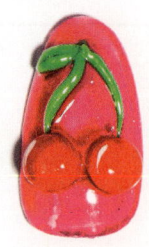
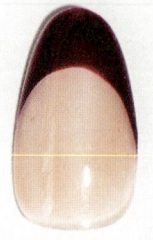
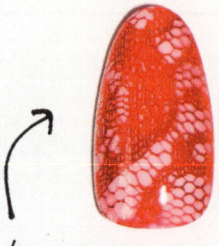

Blooming gel looks are a crowd favourite.

A lace airbrush look works in almost any colour combo.

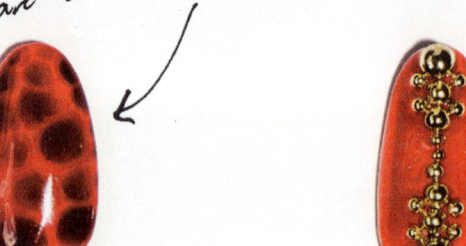
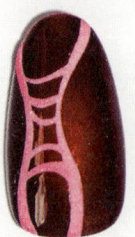

Pearls are one of my go-tos. In my salon they're as much of a staple as rhinestones.

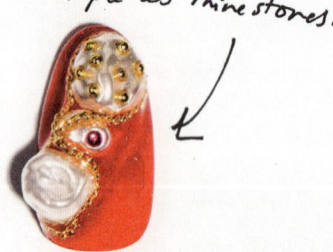
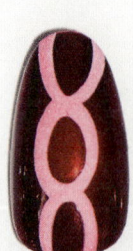
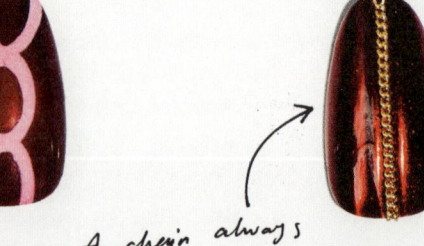

A chain always takes the simplest nail to new heights.

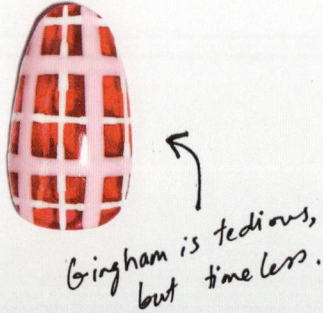
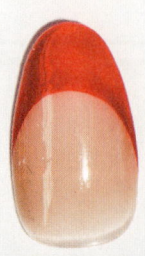
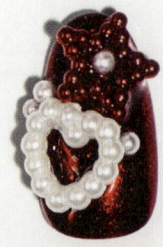

Gingham is tedious, but timeless.

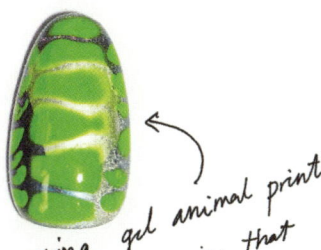
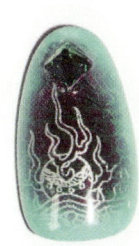
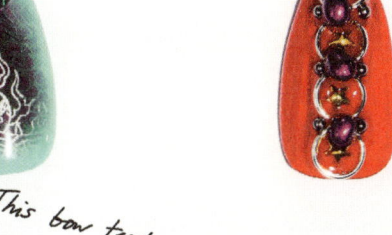

Blooming gel animal prints are another classic that works in every colour.

This bow texture is made from super fine wire and encapsulated in an overlay top coat for a flat finish.

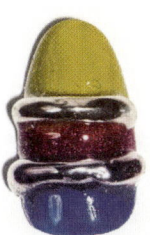
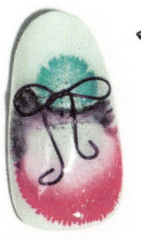
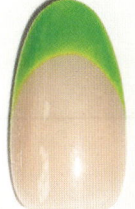

For this one I layered a classic leopard print foil and acrylic flocking.

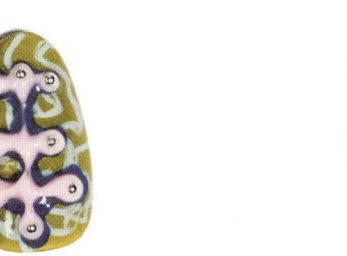
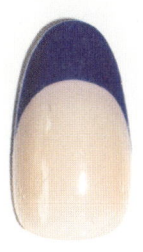
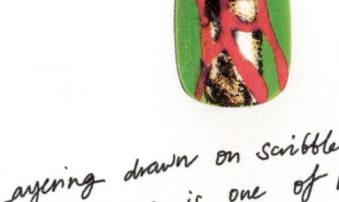

A clear blob gives clients something to run their hands over.

Layering drawn on scribbles with 3D forms is one of my favourite techniques.

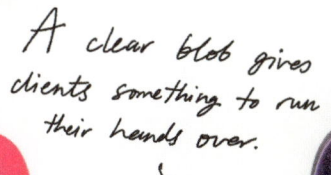
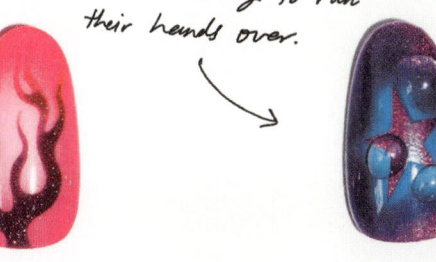
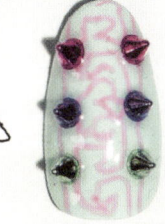

Shell has become a signature in my studio, and I'm not sure I'll ever get sick of it. ↘

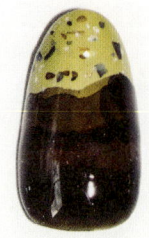
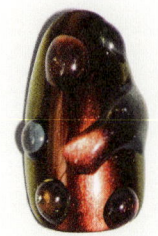

When the big shell pieces don't work the little shell pieces come into play. ↘

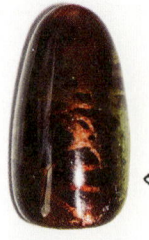
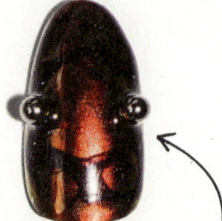

This chrome stamped butterfly never gets old. ↗

Stud piercings on chrome are a simple to do showstopper. ↖

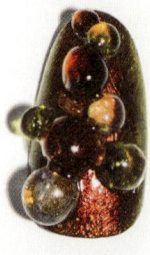
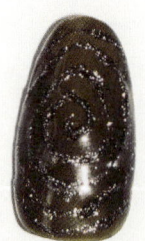
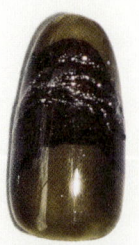

Placing this many studs is time consuming, but the look is unparalleled. ↘

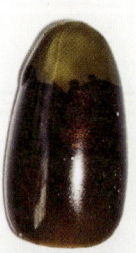
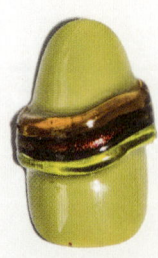
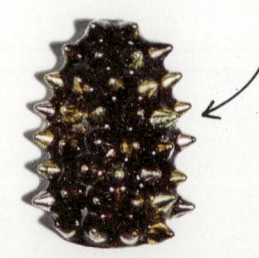

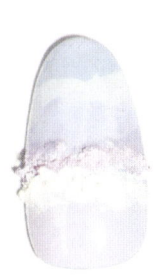 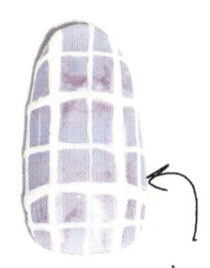 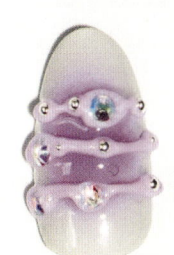

An inlay gingham is another favourite.

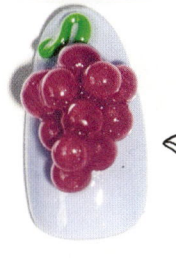 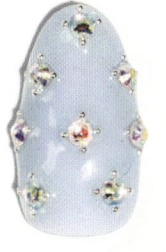

A 3D fruit is the cherry on-top of so many sets (pun intended).

Organic shapes with a touch of chrome are the perfect extension of jewellery on the body.

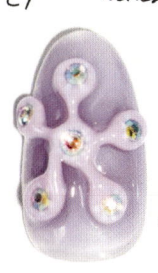 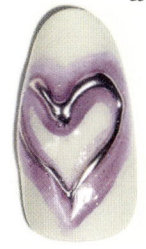

Adding a little sparkle to blobs is a perfect finishing touch.

Textured gel in all forms really came to play on the nails in this set.

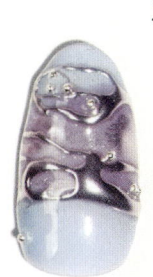 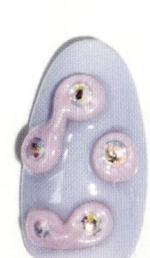 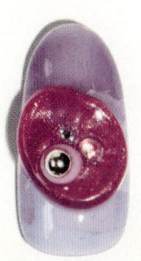

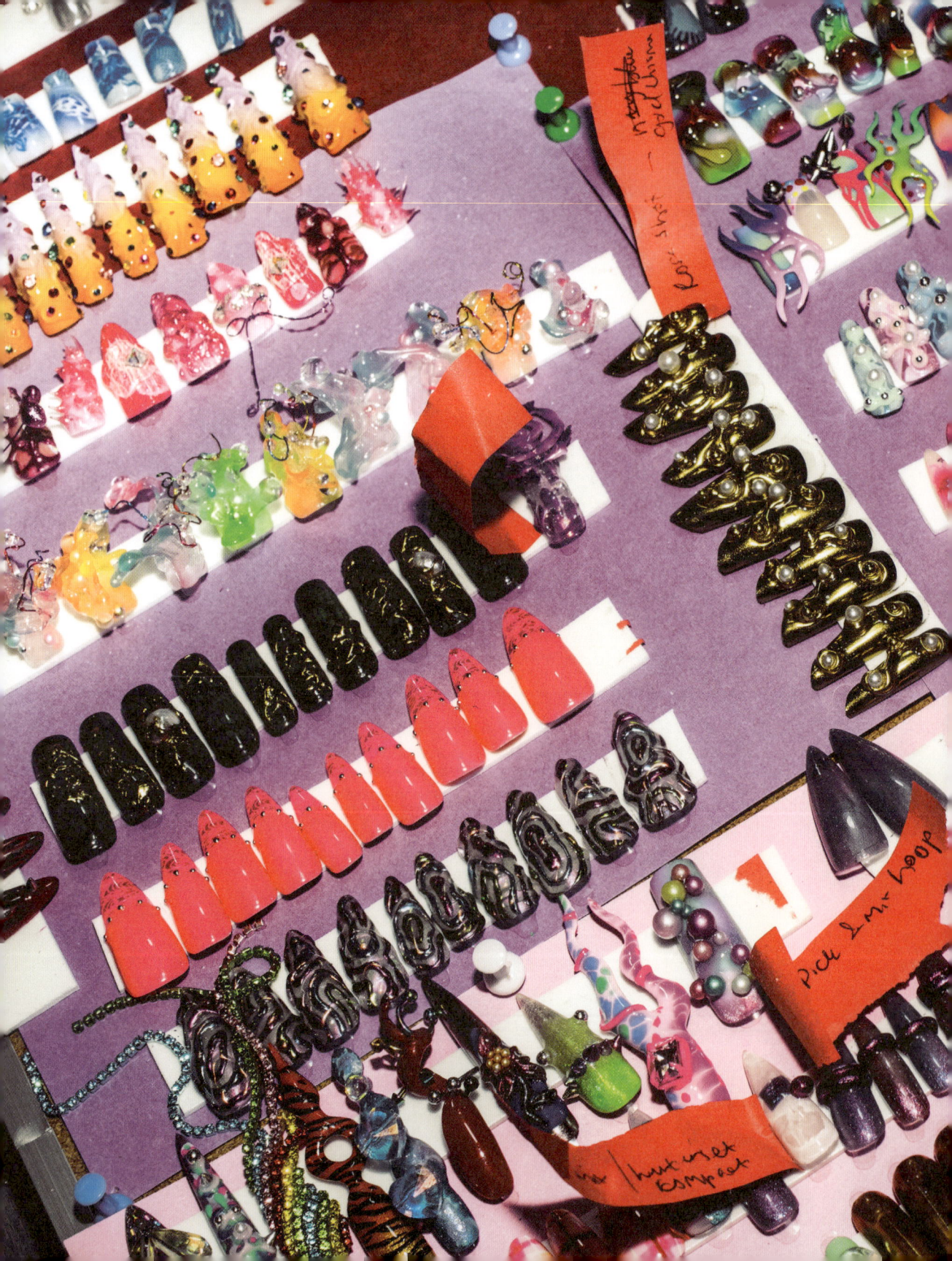

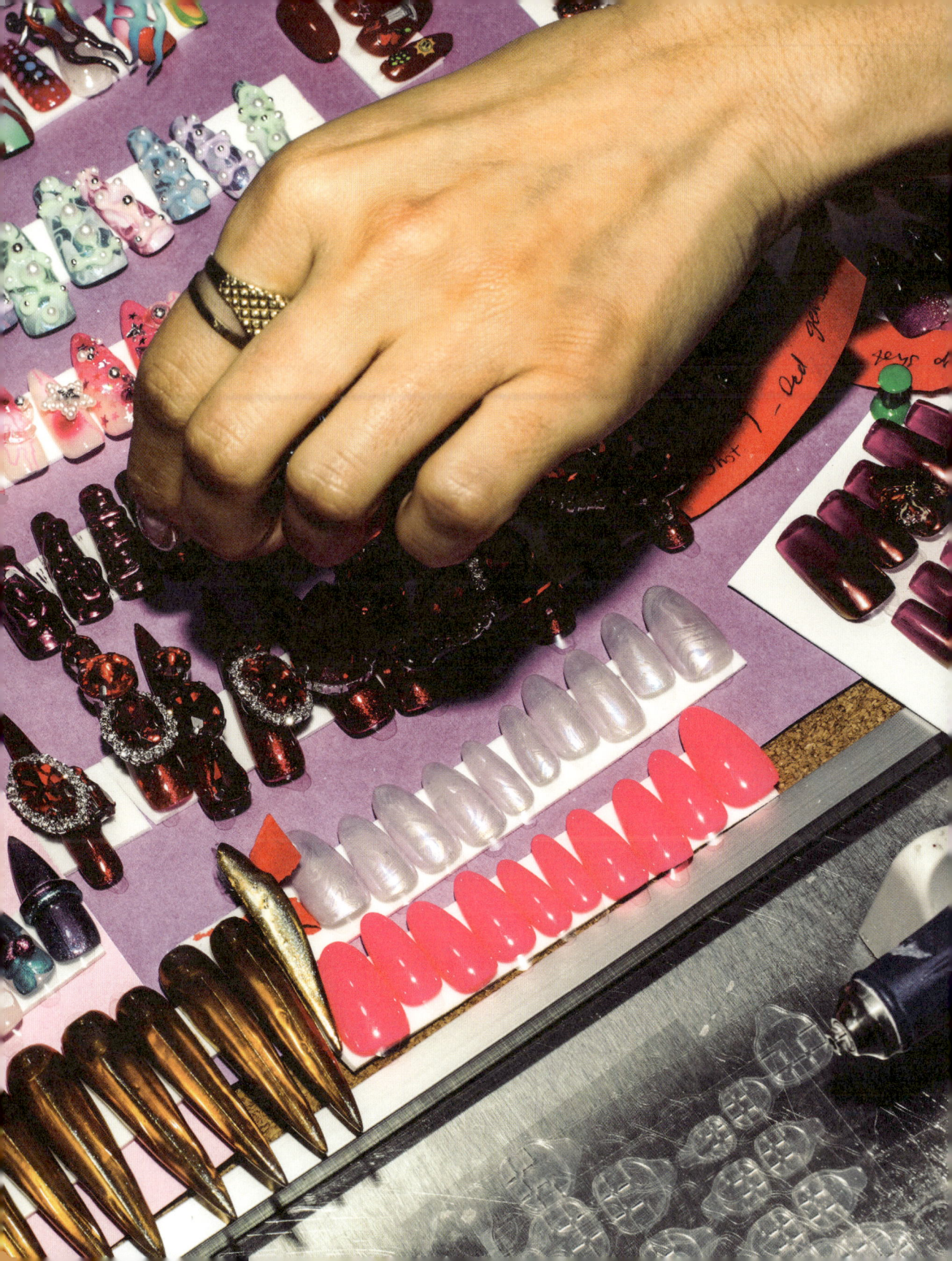

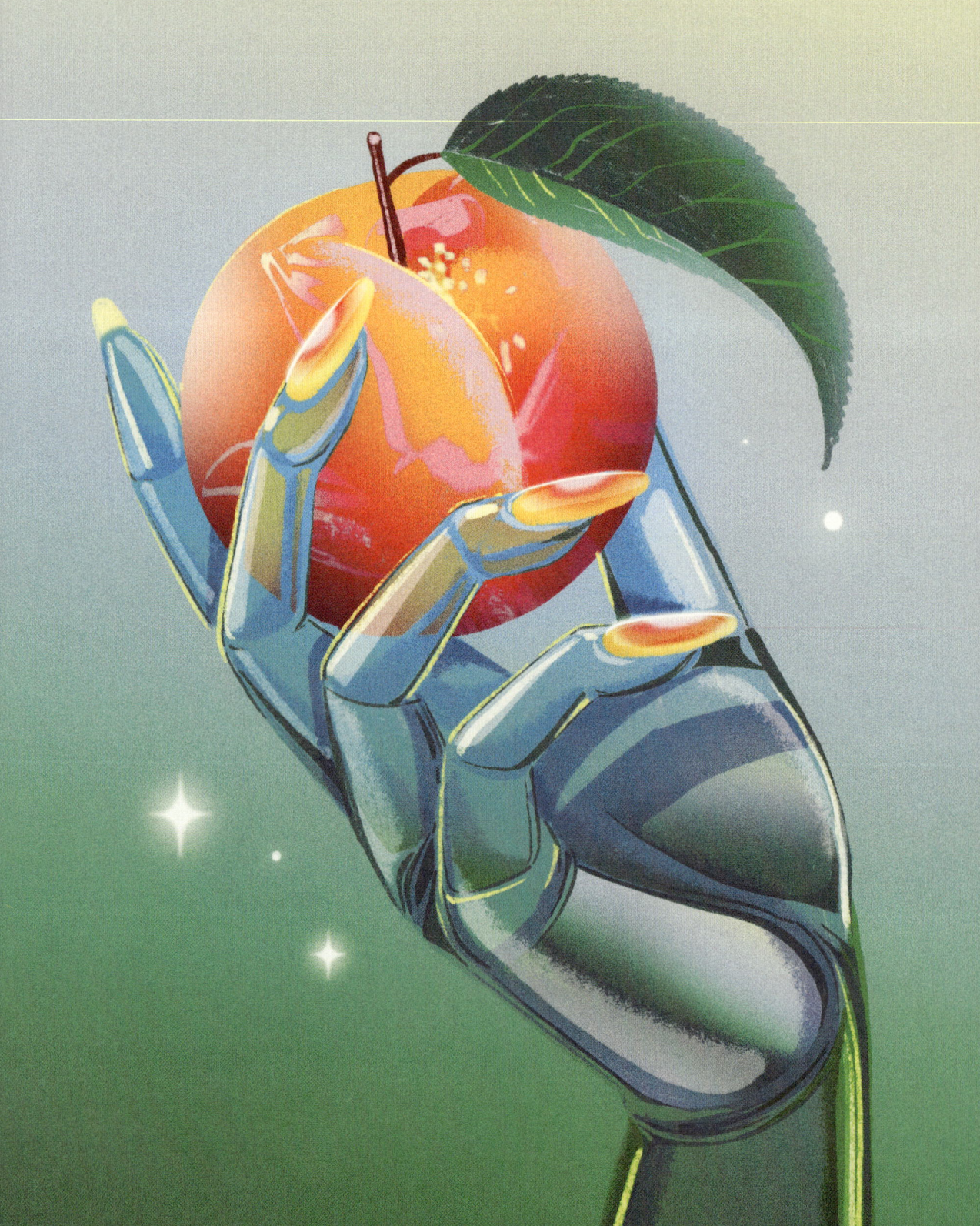

CHAPTER

THE BASICS

THREE

Let's start with the basics

This could be considered the boring part, but I implore you not to turn the page just yet. It isn't like skipping the instructions on a piece of flat pack furniture where, at worst, you might have a rogue screw on the loose. Understanding the basics of nails is the difference between a set that lasts and makes your hands look well-kept or a chipped set and compromised nail health.

It's worth knowing what you're working with. All the DIY pages in this book feature products that anyone can get their hands on. Many nail products however require a license or training, and with good reason, the chemical compounds present in gel and acrylic can cause allergies if used incorrectly. The processes shown in this book are for home care and play, and any nail products that require curing or monomer should be left to the professionals, or you after training if this book inspires it!

With all that in mind, let's do a little background on some of the products, styles and terms used for nail art so when you head to the salon or hold hands with your favourite technician, you know what to ask for. Some of the names and phrases we've grown accustomed to are just plain wrong. Your eponychium is often referred to as the cuticle, shellac is just a branded name for gel colour and BIAB is an acronym for builder in a bottle.

So, if we're going to learn a thing or two about nail art let's get across the basics.

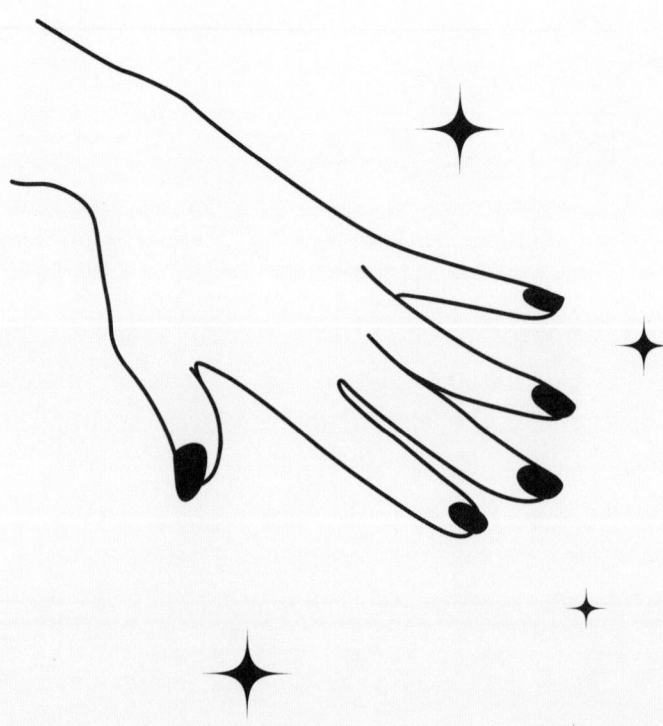

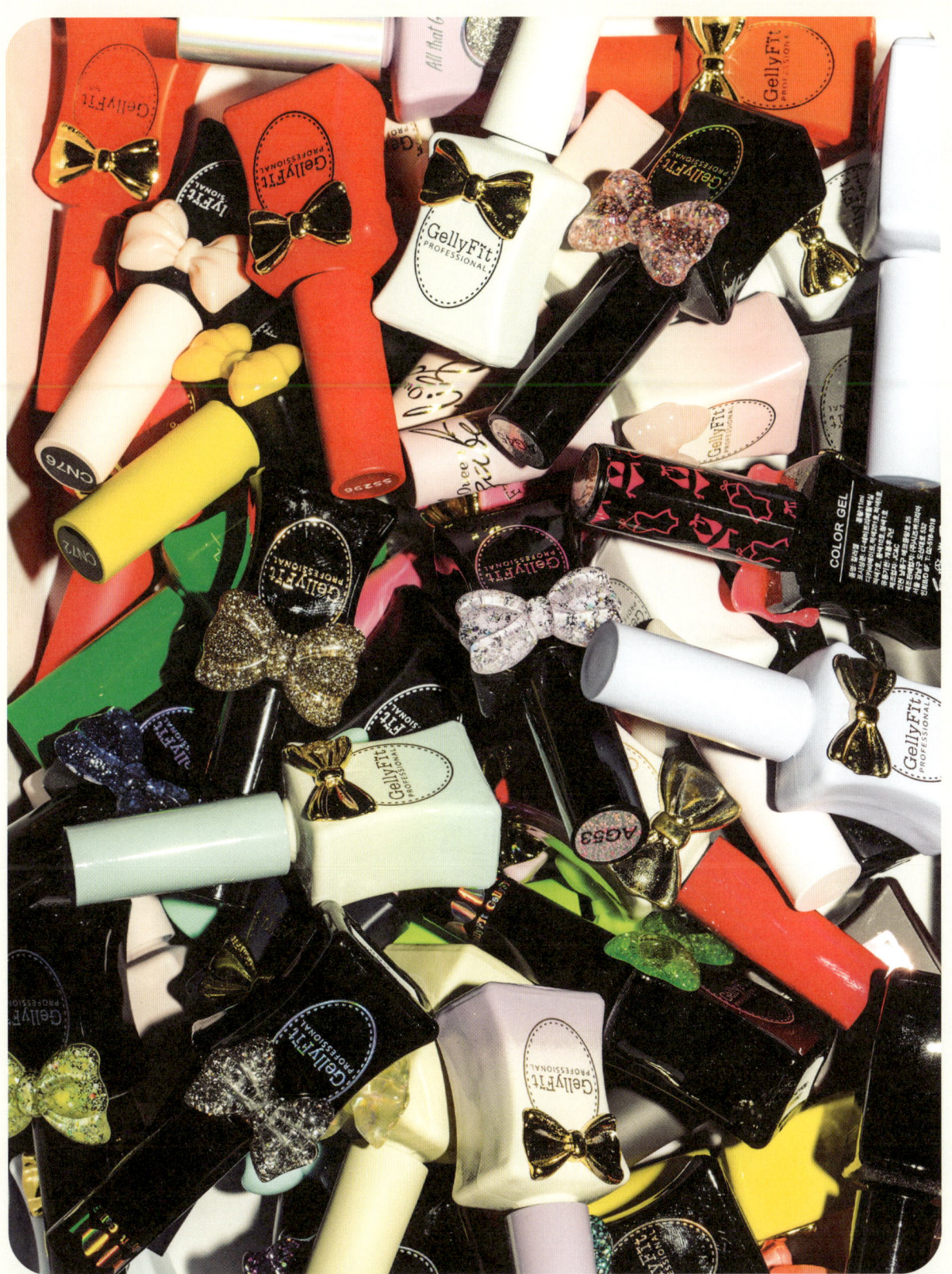

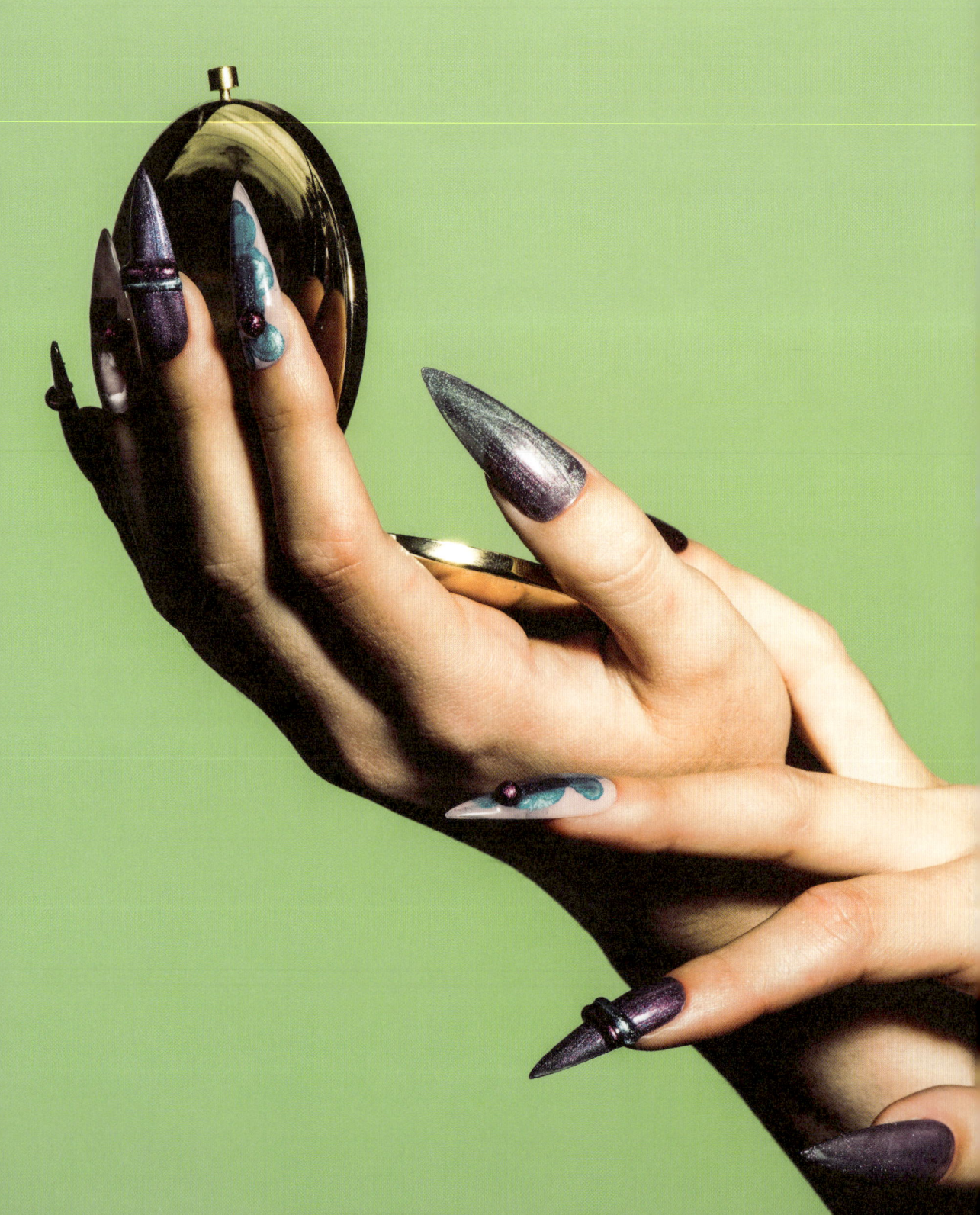

KNOW *Your* NAILS

Everyone's nails look different; there are a few things to understand about the structure of nails to ensure that, no matter what product you use, the health of your nails is maintained.

So what makes up a nail? Let's get into it.

The Nail Plate

THE NAIL PLATE is created in the matrix and is formed by skin cells becoming keratinised. Nails are made up of around 100 layers of compacted keratin cells. Ideal nail plates have a balance between strength and flexibility. Flexibility ensures nails don't crack under pressure or use (jewels not tools!) and strength provides toughness.

This is probably a good time to acknowledge that nails don't 'breathe'. Over filing and poor product removal can damage nails but nail coatings if applied and removed correctly won't damage the nail plate. Be careful not to over file the nail or remove coatings with force. Peeling or flicking off any coating on the nail can damage layers of the nail and compromise the longevity of future sets.

The Side Wall or Lateral Fold

THE SIDE WALL OR LATERAL FOLD acts as a guide for the growth of the nail and protect the nail plate. When filing your nails take extra caution not to file into the side wall. Some nail shapes aren't possible at short lengths. While it can be tempting to taper the nail for a 'slimmer' look, filing past the smile line along the side walls of the nails will cause damage to your nails.

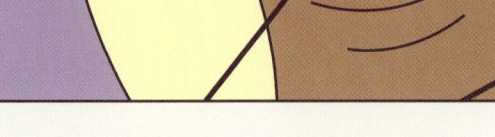

The Cuticle

THE CUTICLE is a thin layer of dead skin that sticks to the nail plate. The cuticle grows with the nail and is formed on the underside of the proximal nail fold. Differentiating the cuticle from the nail plate is often the work of a manicure. When pushed back and softened, the cuticle can be removed from the nail plate. To avoid lifting of any nail coatings, all of the cuticle must be removed from the nail plate. We'll get into the best ways to do that soon so put the nippers down and take a deep breath.

The Eponychium & Proximal Nail Fold

THE PROXIMAL NAIL FOLD is the fold of skin at the base of the nail. The eponychium describes the area that joins the nail plate to the proximal nail fold and protects against bacteria. When doing your manicure, it's important to not break the seal of this area to avoid infections.

The eponychium and proximal nail fold is often mistaken for the cuticle, however this fold is living tissue and should not be cut during a manicure. To tidy the eponychium and prevent it from sticking to the cuticle, regularly apply cream or oil. While it's tempting to cut the cuticle, over time the skin will thicken from scarring.

The Nail Bed

THE NAIL BED is the area underneath your nail that gives it the pink colour. Your nail bed is the shape it is, and if you're a biter, don't fret! The nail bed can extend to the tip of your hyponychium when it's not pushed back. I didn't quite believe it when I was told the same thing by the first nail technician that trained me (thanks Sumi!), I thought she was tricking me to stop me from biting but after maintaining a routine with my manicures, my nail beds look better than ever.

 ## Hot Tip

If you have done a little damage, you can expect the entirety of a nail to grow out in around six months. While everyone's nails grow differently and you can't speed up the process exponentially, stimulating circulation around the matrix by massaging in oil and cream can encourage faster growth. White spots on the nail are a tell-tale sign of damage to the matrix and they will grow out with the nail. Severe damage to the matrix, like blunt force can cause deformities to the nail plate.

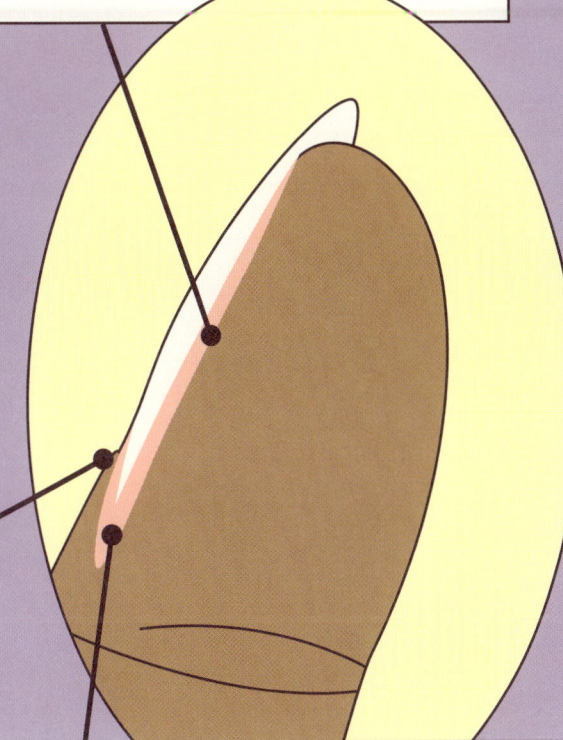

The Hyponychium

THE HYPONYCHIUM is the tissue under the tip of the nail. It acts as a seal to the body and any force to it can lead to a painful break of the seal. When nails are worn long it can naturally extend to support the length of the nail and when nails are worn short it will naturally recede. If it extends, do not push it back or cut it! It's painful and can lead to infection.

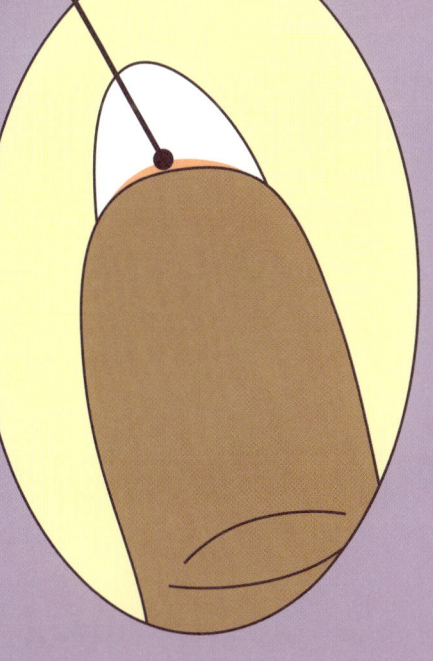

The Matrix

THE MATRIX is directly under the proximal nail fold, this is where the cells that form the nail plate are incubated. The matrix extends from the base of the nail down to the first joint and the length of the matrix determines the thickness of the nail. The longer the matrix, the thicker your nail will be. This is hereditary and no dietary changes will enhance the matrix, however a healthy diet will prevent further weakening of the nails.

SHAPE IT

All nail shapes provide a different look and different wear; everyone has their preference for shape and many techs will offer suggestions around what shapes are most flattering for your hands.

Given nails are a form of self-expression for those who love nail art, I ignore these ideas completely with my clients. The only considerations I take with nail shapes and lengths are my client's lifestyle and condition of the nails. Things I like to consider are occupation, hobbies, sports and any heavy-duty life events like moving home.

Some say shapes that end widest at the tip are the most complimentary on wider fingers, whereas tapered shapes work best with slender fingers. These ideas are based on balancing the look of the width of the fingers with the width of the tip of the nail. There are many rules and preferences taught about the lengths and shapes of nails. While they have their merit in a traditional manicure, and there are some rules in place to ensure the health of the nail, no two clients are the same. This is where consulting with a client on their lifestyle is crucial.

The only time it's best to reconsider a shape is if that natural length of your nail will not support the silhouette. If your nails are short and you want to achieve a stiletto shape, there's a possibility of filing into the side wall to taper the nail into a point. To avoid damage and weakening of the nail bed this is a hard no go!

With that in mind, let's look at some nail shapes.

NAIL Shapes

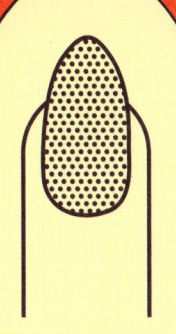 ALMOND

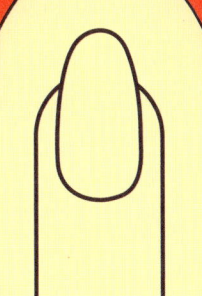 OVAL

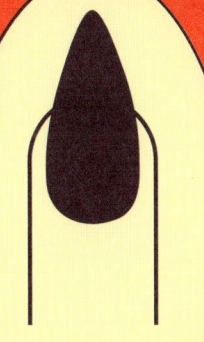 STILETTO

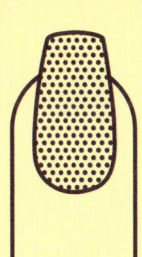 SQUARE

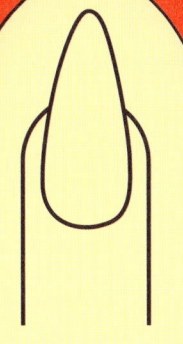 RUSSIAN STILETTO

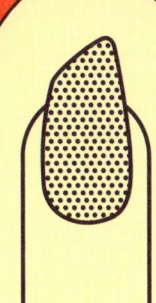 LIPSTICK

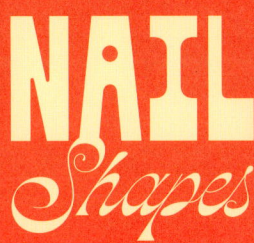 SQUOVAL

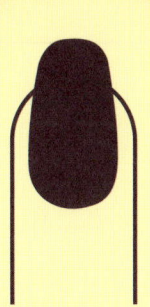

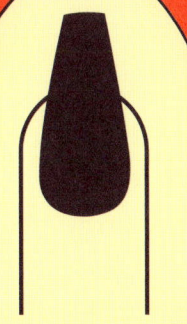 COFFIN

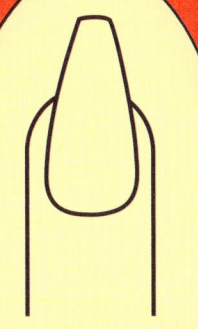 BALLERINA

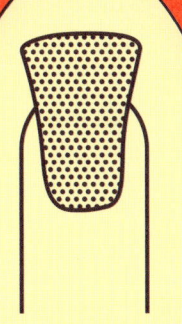 DUCK

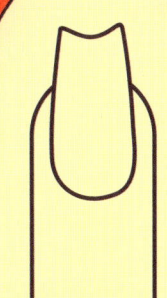 CONCAVE

PAINT IT

There are so many products that can be used in a manicure, let's break down some of the most common.

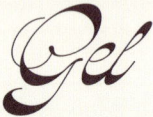

Nail polish

A varnish with a thin consistency that air dries and can be removed with acetone or nail polish remover.

Gel

Gel comes in many different consistencies and has many uses but let's start with regular gel colours. Normally they're soft gels which means they can be soaked off once the topcoat has been filed away. Gel colours are often referred to as shellac, however that is just one brand's name for the product. Gels must be applied thinly and evenly to ensure the curing process is uninterrupted.

Gel has photo initiators which react to UV light. When this happens the gel hardens and with all gels that don't feature a non-wipe finish, the gel with have an inhibition layer on top which leaves the gel sticky until wiped with isopropyl alcohol or top coated.

★ HOT TIP ★

All nail coverings can cause damage if the nail is over filed in preparation or if the coating is removed incorrectly. The metro card flick, teeth pull and gel peel are all ways of forcing or pulling the coating which will inevitably remove layers of your nail with the product which will compromise your nail health. Repeated skin contact with uncured gel can cause allergic reactions so careful application is necessary.

Builder gel or overlay gel

Both builder gels and overlay gels have a thicker consistency made for adding strength to the manicure. While these products can't chemically make your nails stronger, the thick coating does inhibit the amount of wear and tear your nails are exposed to over the span of your manicure. BIAB refers to builder in a bottle and can come in a variety of colours. The purpose being to cut down application time and maintain a neat grow out. Builder gels come in both hard and soft gel formulas. Hard gels must be filed off while soft gels can be soaked off.

ACRYLIC

What we generally refer to as acrylics are enhancements made of a mix of monomer liquids and polymer powders. The application of acrylic nails requires dipping a brush from monomer liquids into polymer powders, the pairing of the two, when exposed to air, begins to harden. Acrylic can be applied as an overlay or over glued on tips and forms, it also comes in a variety of colours making it popular for use in creating 3D art. Acrylic can be filed and soaked off in acetone.

HOT TIP

Acrylic in the nail industry, like gel was originally derived from the dental industry however MMA is no longer recommended for use, with EMA being the preferred monomer.

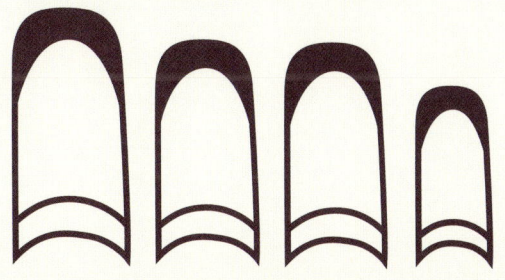

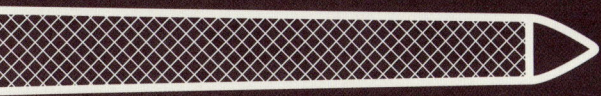

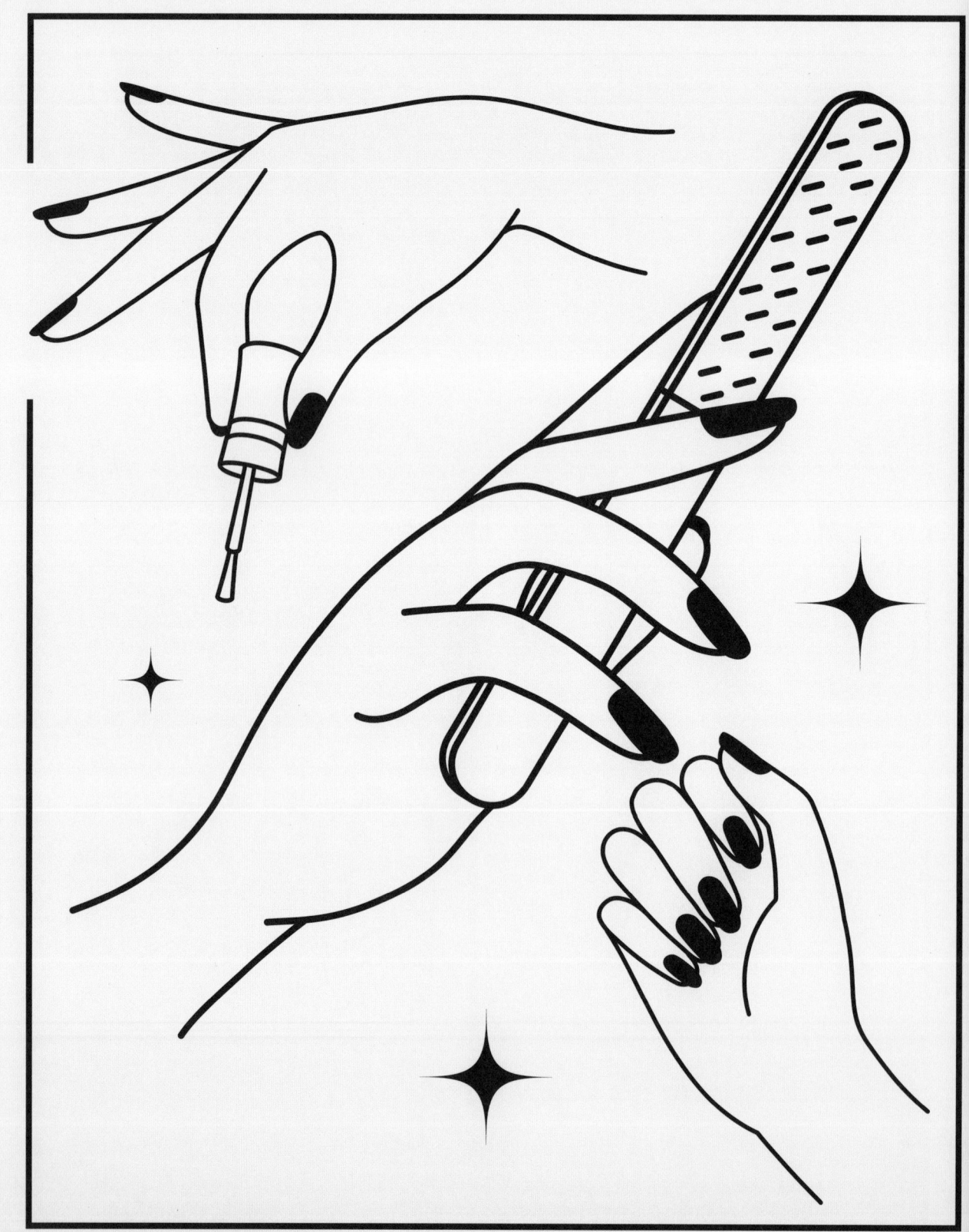

ACRYLGEL OR POLYGEL

As the name suggests acrylgel is the love child of acrylic and gel. It is made to be as hard after curing as acrylic, but as flexible as gel to ensure strength and durability. They can come in tube form or tub form and must be cured with UV or LED lights to harden. It can be used to both create extensions or form a strong overlay on a natural nail. Polygel is similar but can be soaked off in acetone while acrylgel must be filed down first.

HOT TIP

Nail enhancements are designed to be worn no longer than 3-4 weeks. While many sets may last longer, structure-built sets that use either gel or acrylic are generally sculpted with an apex in mind. The apex is the highest point on the nail when you view your set from the side. The apex holds the most product, it sits on the lower third of the nail bed on a short to medium length and on the middle part on a long set. It is designed to balance the weight of the tip of the nail so that, as your nail grows, the tip isn't as likely to break under pressure. As nails grow out, this apex is pushed further up the nail bed towards the tip and the structure of your set is compromised.

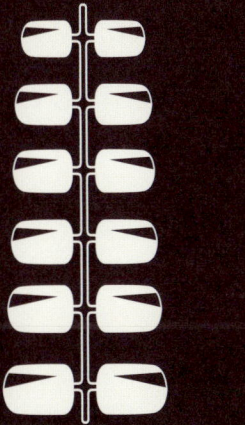

Full over gel extension

The full cover gel extension spans from cuticle to tip. They're applied using an extension gel rather than glue and they come in a variety of shapes and structures making them perfect for clients who love to change the shape of their sets frequently. Full cover gel extensions can be soaked off in acetone.

FIBRE GEL OR FIBREGLASS GEL

Fibre gel is designed to emulate the structure of the natural nail. With microfibres in the gel, this gel is designed to withstand the pressure of wear and tear in similar ways to the natural nail. Some brands even have colours that look just like the natural nail, making them perfect for fixing breaks or cracks in the nail. They can also be used to extend the nail.

Silk wraps

Much like fibre gel, silk wraps can emulate the structure of the natural nail with a woven texture that holds flexibility. Silk wraps can be used to 'band-aid' a tear in the nail. This is especially useful if a split is on the nail bed rather than the free edge and can ensure the split doesn't worsen with time. Silk wraps can also be used to create extensions when encapsulated in gel.

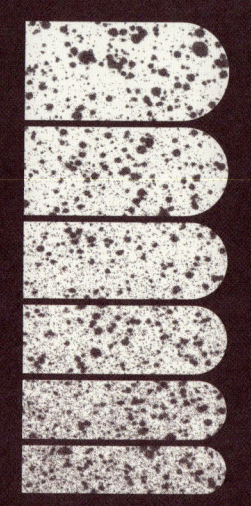

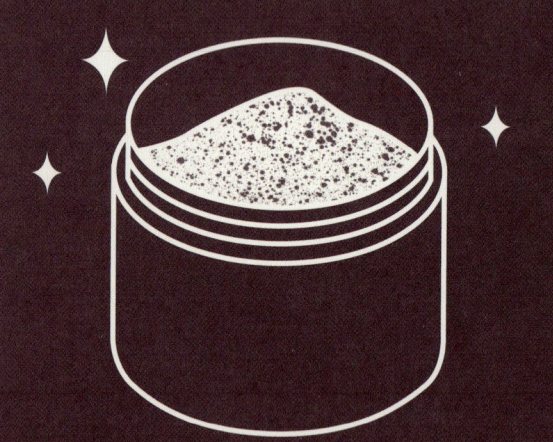

Dip powder

Dip powder, like acrylic, hardens when exposed to air and uses acrylic powder, however the liquid that forms the bond and hardening is cyanoacrylate, a resin-like glue. While dip powder can be hard wearing, it can lack flexibility.

Forms

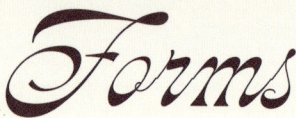

Forms are sticker like guides that sit under the free edge of the nail and are used as a removable base for techs to build out extensions. They're ideal for repairing breaks or extending nails into any shape. Any gels that are strong enough to add structure like hard gel, builder gel or polygel are great to use with forms.

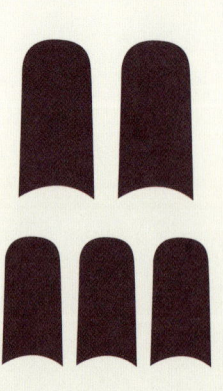

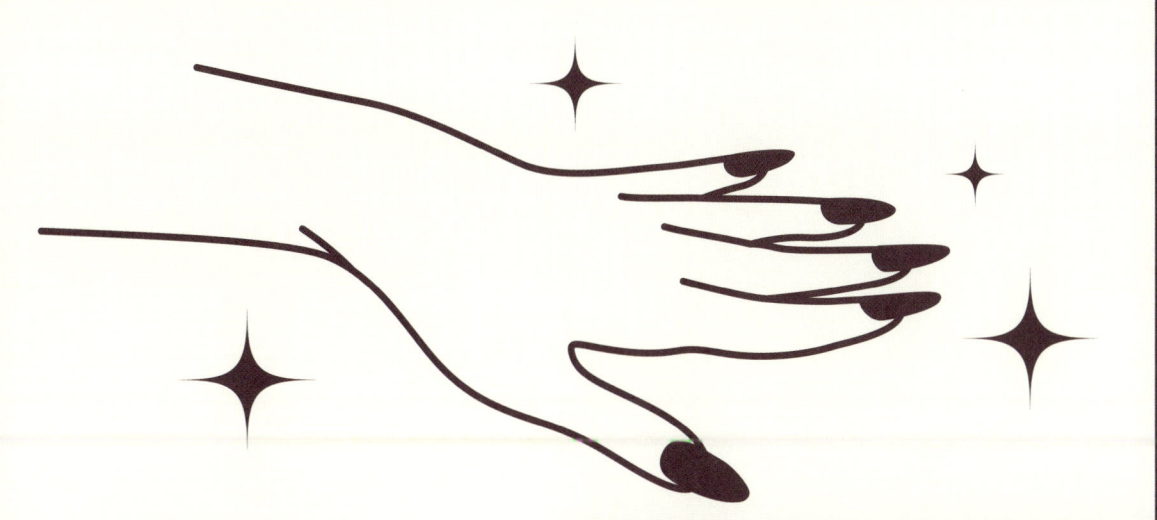

DUAL FORMS

Dual forms perform much the same function as forms however rather than building on top of the free edge, dual forms require product to be applied onto a form that is then pressed onto the nail and flash cured into position. Once it's attached the nail must be fully cured and the tech will carefully remove the dual form from the nail. Gels that are strong enough to add structure can be used with dual forms however super viscous and self-leveling gels are not suitable as they tend to run with the pressure of gravity once the dual form is pressed onto the nail.

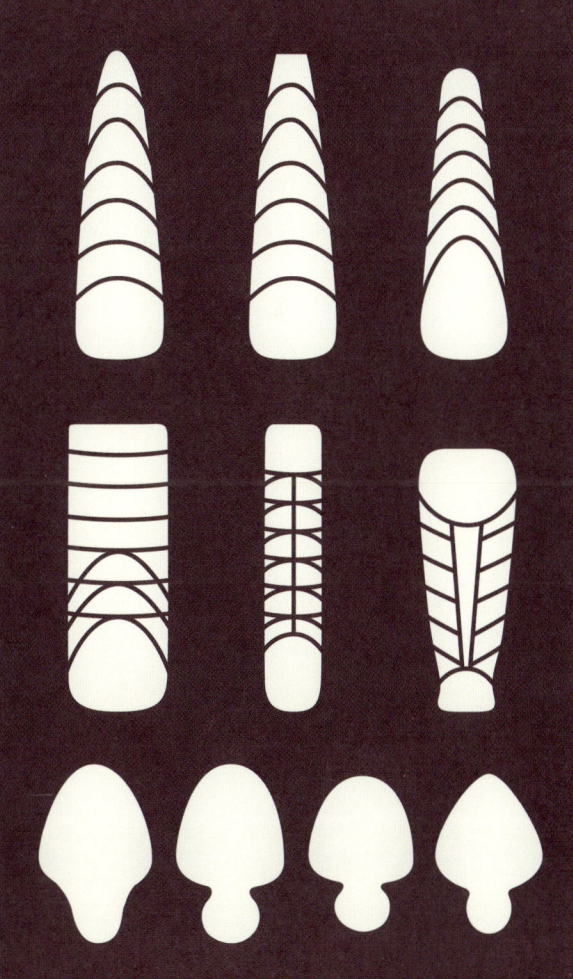

AT *Home* TOOLKIT

If you're going to be looking after your nails at home, these are the main tools you'll need to have handy.

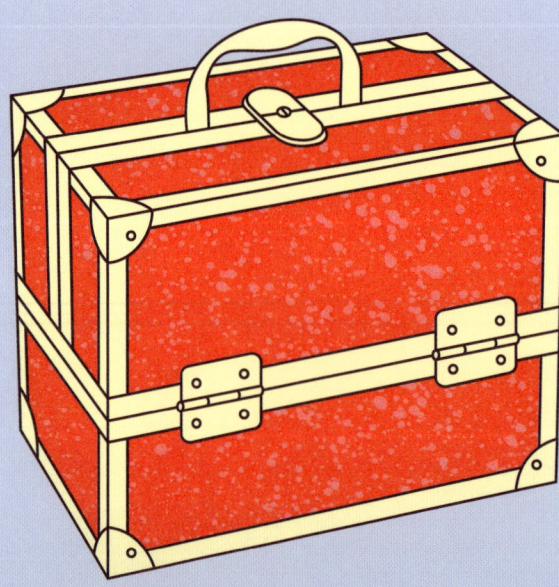

1
Orange wood sticks or a cuticle pusher

These are a necessity for pushing back the cuticle to reveal the full length of the nail bed and tidy up the nail prior to applying any coatings.

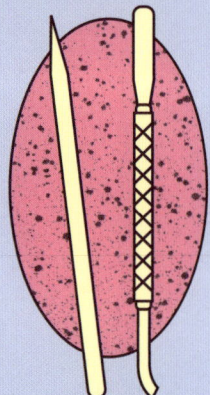

2
Nail file

Nail file grits are organised in much the same way as sandpaper, the higher the number, the finer the grit. Nothing coarser than 180 grit should be used on the natural nail. My preference for natural nails is 180 grit or higher, my personal favourite for filing and shaping natural nails is 240.

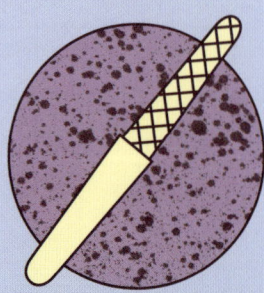

3
Nail buffer

I love a natural buff and shine so buffers with a super smooth side are my favourite. Super fine buffers are most often available in a 600/4,000 grit block. They're a staple for adding shine to the natural nail and have great skin polishing benefits that we'll get into in the DIY manicure.

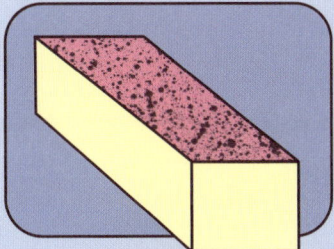

4
Cuticle nippers

Cuticle nippers must be used with extreme caution! It doesn't take much to nip away live skin so follow the steps provided in the manicure section of this book to ensure you don't cause more harm than good. In saying that, the only thing more precarious than using cuticle nippers, is using dull cuticle nippers so ensure you always store yours with the cap on!

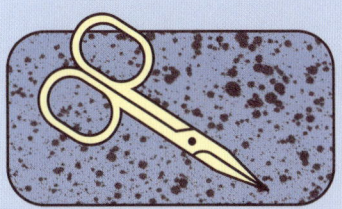

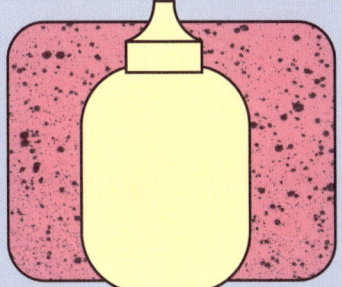

5
Cuticle remover

This magical liquid is going to remove all the dead skin cells from your nail plate, which helps any nail coating last as long as possible. Ensure you remove the cuticle remover and wash your hands thoroughly once you finish tidying up your cuticles. Cuticle remover makes the cuticle very soft and spongy so move slowly when taking nippers to the cuticle to avoid tearing.

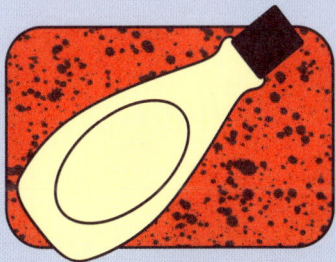

6
Nail polish remover

This is a necessity for removing old nail product. If you're using regular nail polish, acetone free nail polish remover is suitable however if you're removing gel, acrylic or extensions of any sort, you'll need acetone.

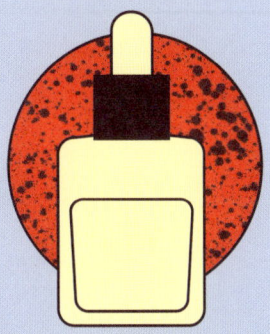

7
Cuticle oil

Cuticle oil should be used to hydrate the nails and cuticle area as frequently as possible, in an ideal world, you'd reapply cuticle oil as often as you wash your hands!

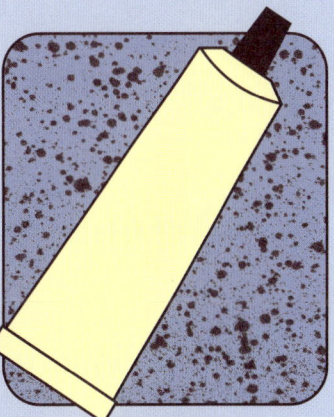

8
Hand cream

Lather up your hands frequently to keep you skin supple, this makes future manicures neater and easier.

AT HOME CARE

If you have coatings on your nails, keep it simple. Lather your cuticles in cuticle oil, not once a week but as many times a day as you remember to! Treat it like you would lip balm. Think about how little you moisturise your hands but how often you wash them, that's how frequently we're stripping the natural oils from our hands. Good spots to keep a cuticle oil include, but are not limited to, your handbag, your desk, your bedside table and your car.

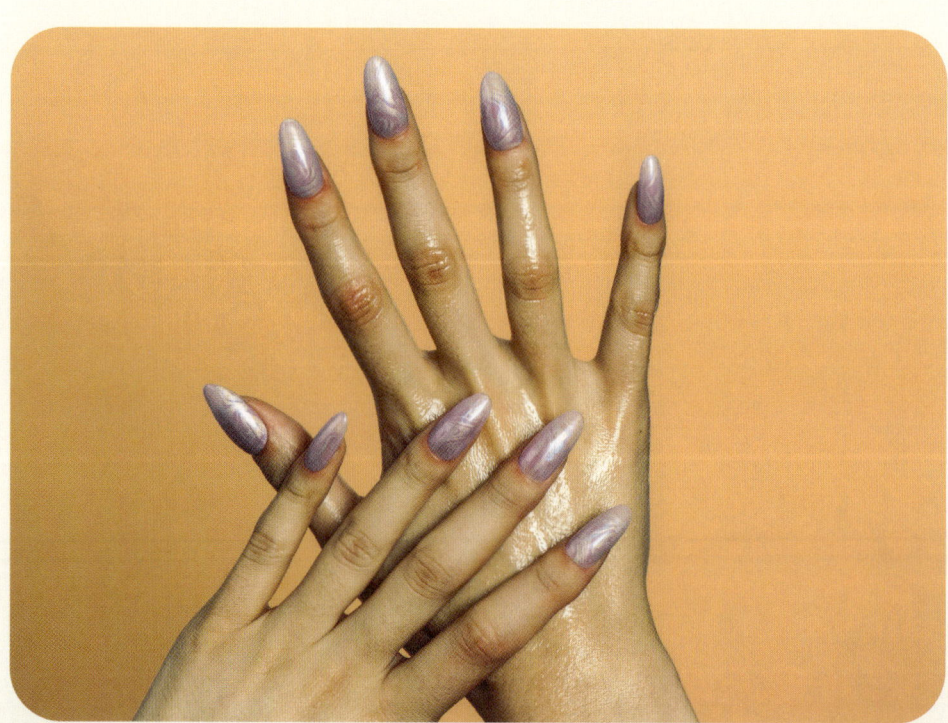

Mannequin Hands

Maintaining the health of your nails when wearing coatings includes things as simple as maintaining the recommended wear time as suggested by your nail technician. Technicians will recommend anywhere between 2-4-week cycles depending on the nail coating, length of your nails and lifestyle. It is professional guidance to ensure that the weight distribution on your nails isn't likely to lead to weakness in the nail bed and painful breaks.

What if I've broken a nail?

Whatever you do, avoid taking a file to your nails while you have a coating on. While sometimes it can be necessary if you've split your nail, be careful not to file into the side wall trying to file the length of the split. It's important not to push your file into the space where your nail plate ends and your skin begins on the sides of your nails. Filing into the side wall to stop a nail from splitting further or pushing your file into this space in the hopes of tapering the nail for a 'thinner' appearance causes long-term damage. It'll cause separation between the nail bed and the nail plate and cause more weakness in the most vulnerable part of the nail.

Taping or bandaging the nail until it can be fixed is ideal. Applying super glue, nail glue or wearing band aids for extensive lengths of time can lead to trapping liquid between the nail plate and the coating which can leave your nail susceptible to infections, most commonly pseudomonas aka 'greenies'. A pseudomonas nail infection is caused by a common bacteria called pseudomonas aeruginosa and the waste of the bacteria causes a green hue on the nail bed.

If a break is causing disruption to your lifestyle, book in as quickly as possible to have your nail repaired. If it's a state of emergency and is catching, cut the length of any extensions to avoid further pressure or uneven weight distribution on the nail bed. You can then carefully file off the top coat and soak off the remaining coating in acetone. If your nail is tender or bleeding avoid removing the coating until you've consulted a professional.

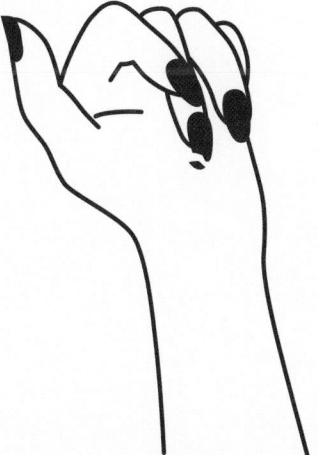

Salon FAQs

> Now for some answers to questions that might pop into your head during a nail service.

Why do the tools come in that sterilisation pouch?

Depending on which country and even city you get your nails done in, the requirements vary. If you're somewhere that requires sterilisation, any tools that touch skin should come in sterilisation pouches where a colour change marker will let you know that the pouch has been through a cycle in the autoclave. The autoclave kills harmful bacteria, fungi, and viruses using steam in a pressure vessel. In some places disinfection is the only legal requirement, that process involves cleaning tools in ideally a hospital grade disinfectant – think of your classic Barbicide and the like.

The difference between disinfecting and sterilising? Disinfecting kills most germs while sterilising kills all microorganisms. The combination of both is ideal to minimise the risk of infections. All porous materials used in the service like orange wood sticks and nail files should be disposed of.

Why do some manicures cost different amounts?

This one has a range of answers but mainly it comes down to the service provided. Contributing factors can be the cost and quality of products used during the service and the cost of running a business in the area you're in. Independent nail technicians aren't under the time constraints of walk-in salons so they can provide services that take more time and can charge more. Shopping centre salons are expected to service walk-in clients and have tighter time constraints per service meaning the profit margins differ.

Why does my nail tech flip my hand upside-down sometimes?

If you're getting a builder gel manicure or an overlay on top of your set, your nail tech might ask you to flip your hand over. This is a quick way to ensure the gel is perfectly level and the highest point of the overlay is right where the apex should be on your nail. Gel continues to move until the curing process is complete so checking that the gel is applied to support an apex for strength and has a smooth rather than lumpy appearance is imperative. Flipping the hand and touching over the nail with a detail brush is an easy and effective way to do so.

Why do some gel products get hot when curing?

Heat is released as gel hardens and cures under LED or UV light. Often the layer of gel is thin and therefore doesn't heat up as much. However, when the gel has a thick consistency or is applied in a thick layer, this chemical process can be felt, this is called a heat spike. Other factors like damage to the natural nail or the proximity to certain points in the hormonal cycle can impact the severity of this feeling. It's best to remove your hand from exposure to the lamp until the heat spike subsides.

Are nail lamps safe for frequent use?

The studies on this vary and it's important to consider whether brands or companies have had a hand in the research being conducted when consuming this information. As time passes and technology shifts the conversations we have around the safety of UV and LED lamps will continue to change. What we do know for sure is that UV energy's harm is dependent on wavelength, duration and frequency of exposure and intensity. All types of nail lamps emit UVA energy as this is the wavelength capable of curing UV nail gel products. The amount of UV you're exposed to while getting your nails done is equal to spending a couple of minutes in the sun each day between appointments.

Should I wear sunscreen when I go to the nail salon?

While protecting your skin from exposure of UV rays is helpful in every setting, it is important for the adhesion of your nail coatings that oils aren't present on the nail bed before a manicure. If you apply sunscreen to your hands, allow enough time for it to be soaked in so the oils don't compromise the adhesion of your set. Another alternative is to wear UV resistant gloves with the tips exposed.

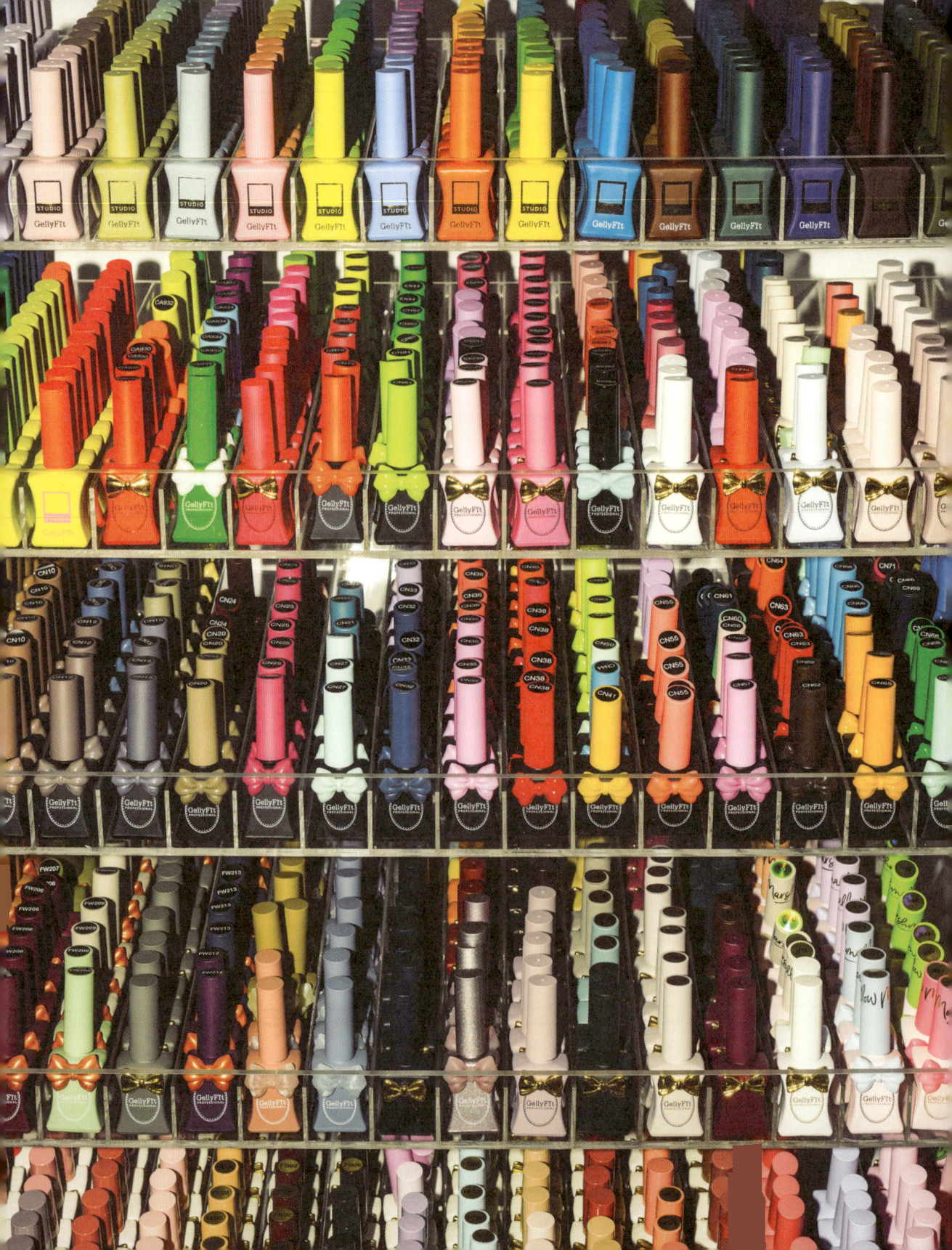

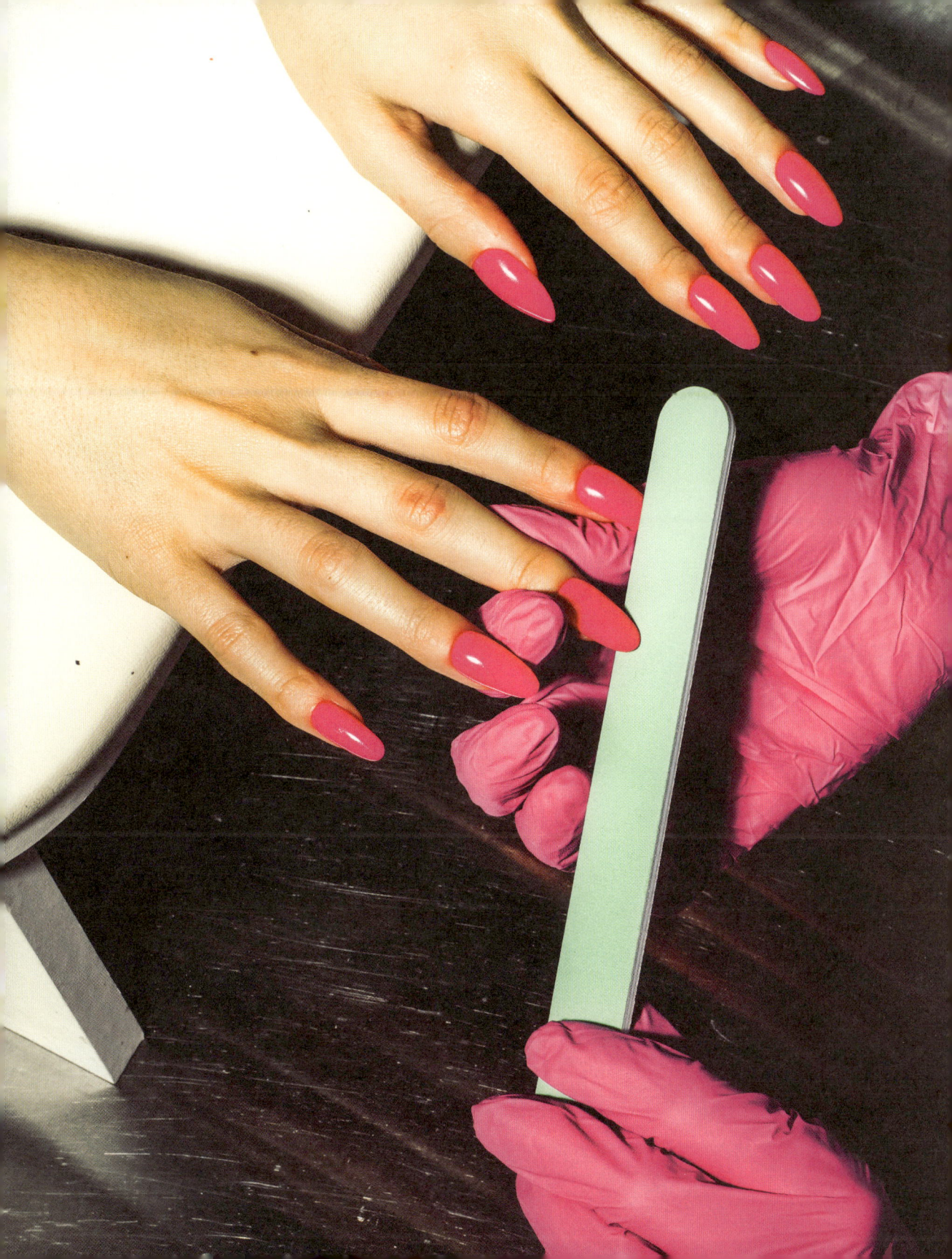

Why can't I touch anything during a nail appointment?

There are a few reasons so let's break this down:

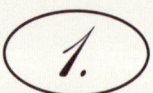

Between shaping and buffing the nail and the application of a base your nail technician will wipe the nail with a prep liquid or isopropyl alcohol to ensure the nail coating adheres to the nail. Oil, dust or liquids on the nail plate can ruin the adhesion of the nail coating. Touching your hair or skin can leave oil on the nail plate while tapping your phone or touching other surfaces can leave the nail plate dusty.

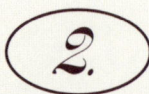

The same applies after the application of the nail coating, if any nail coating that needs to be cured has been applied then the texture on the nail is extremely sticky as a result of the inhibition layer. This must be cleaned off with alcohol before touching anything including your skin. Excess exposure to the skin can lead to possible allergies and dust attaching to the surface of the nail can lead to a messy final look.

Your nail technician could be painting something with an extremely fine brush or working with a product that is fast levelling, meaning it moves constantly until cured. The chances for product to get damaged is high. Movements that you would deem minute or only slight, are huge on the hand. Things as simple as brushing your hair away from your face using your shoulder forces your hand to move drastically. These movements can cause issues for how long your set lasts or can expose your skin to products only designed for the nail plate.

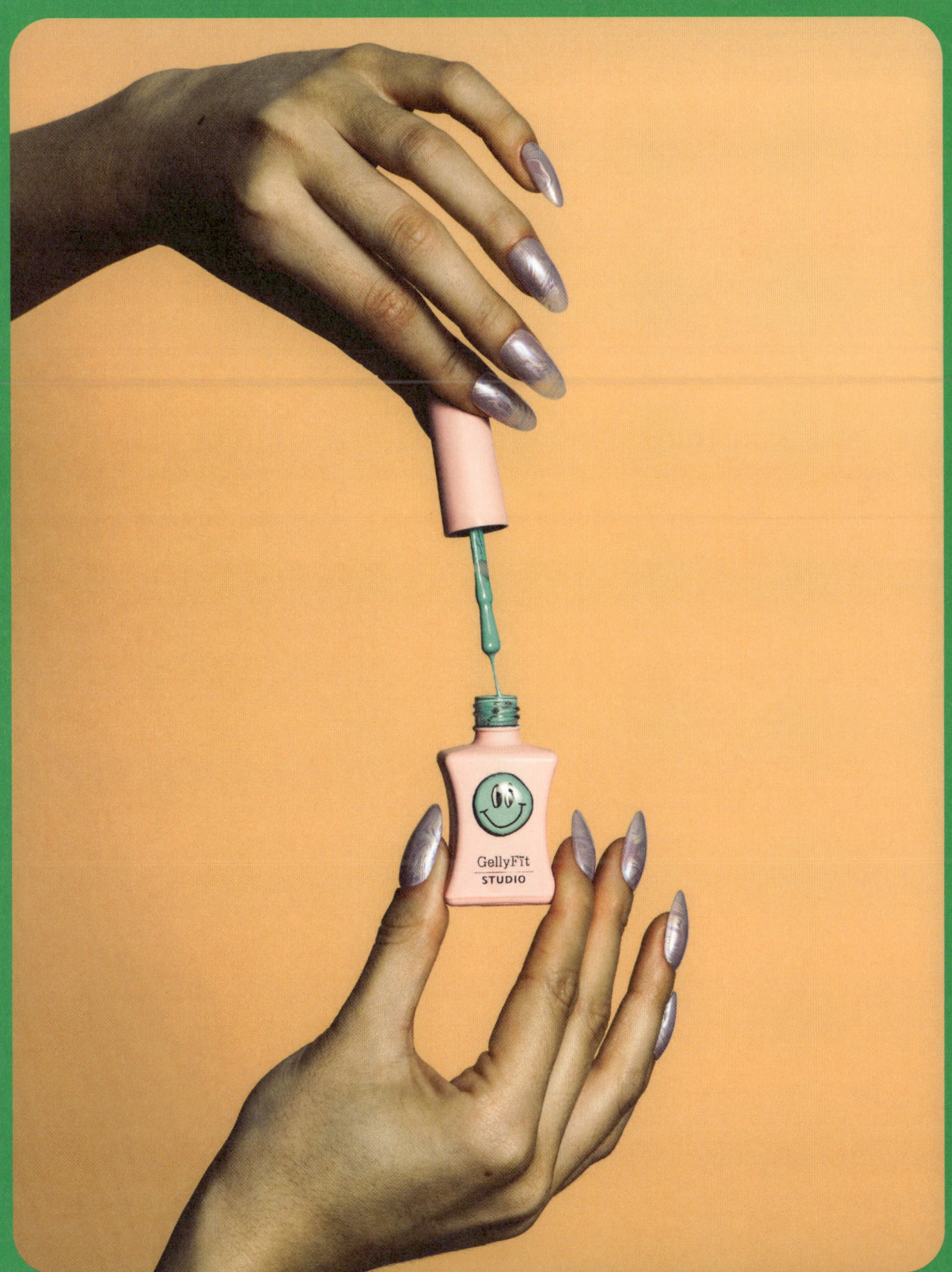

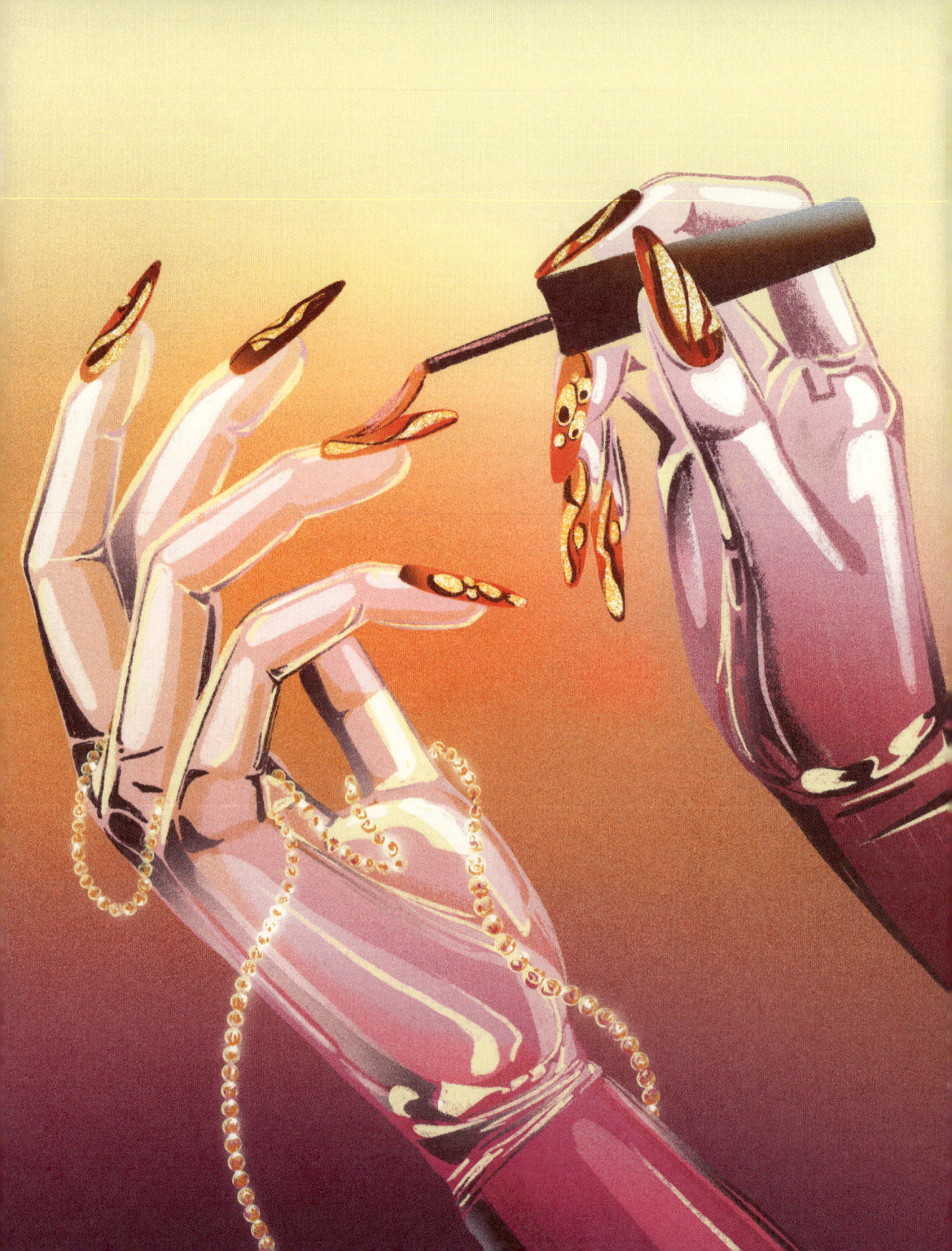

CHAPTER

HANDS-ON TUTORIALS

FOUR

◆

𝓐s with all art, once you get the medium down pat you can really let your creativity flow. This section is all about how to do it yourself, from a proper manicure, to filing and even painting your own sets. There are a million ways to DIY, but I've made sure to use products that anyone can get their hands on.

    We're about to run through the basics of an at home manicure. Many of the ways we do a manicure in the salon have changed, with that in mind we've altered the manicure process to best reflect the process we use to achieve a neat and tidy base, ready for art. There are tips and tricks for making your nails neat and presentable, and some home care and maintenance tips to keep your hands looking like a mannequin's.

    So steady your hand and let's get started!

Manicure

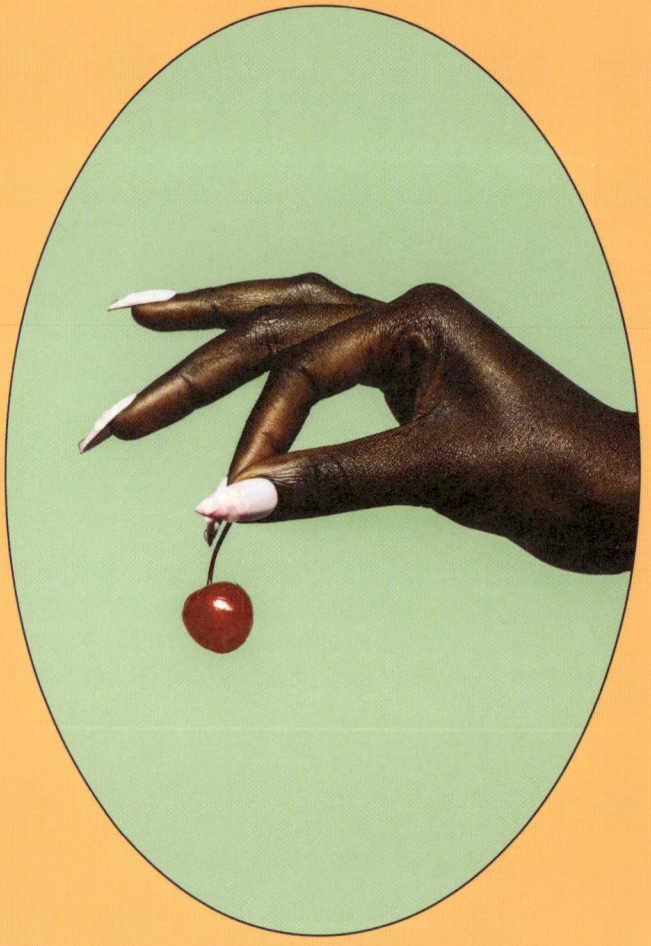

For those who love to indulge in a bit of self-care from time to time, or even for those who just love a natural nail, let's get into the best ways to manage your own nails. An at home manicure can achieve beautiful results, I'm talking great shape, great shine and cute art with nail polish alone.

Plenty of the tips and tricks from the salon can be added to your home routine for a perfect finish. Manicures have shifted exponentially in the last 20 years and some of the classic means of removing cuticle from the nail bed and prepping the nail have changed. Today we're going for the safest, simplest and most effective at home manicure.

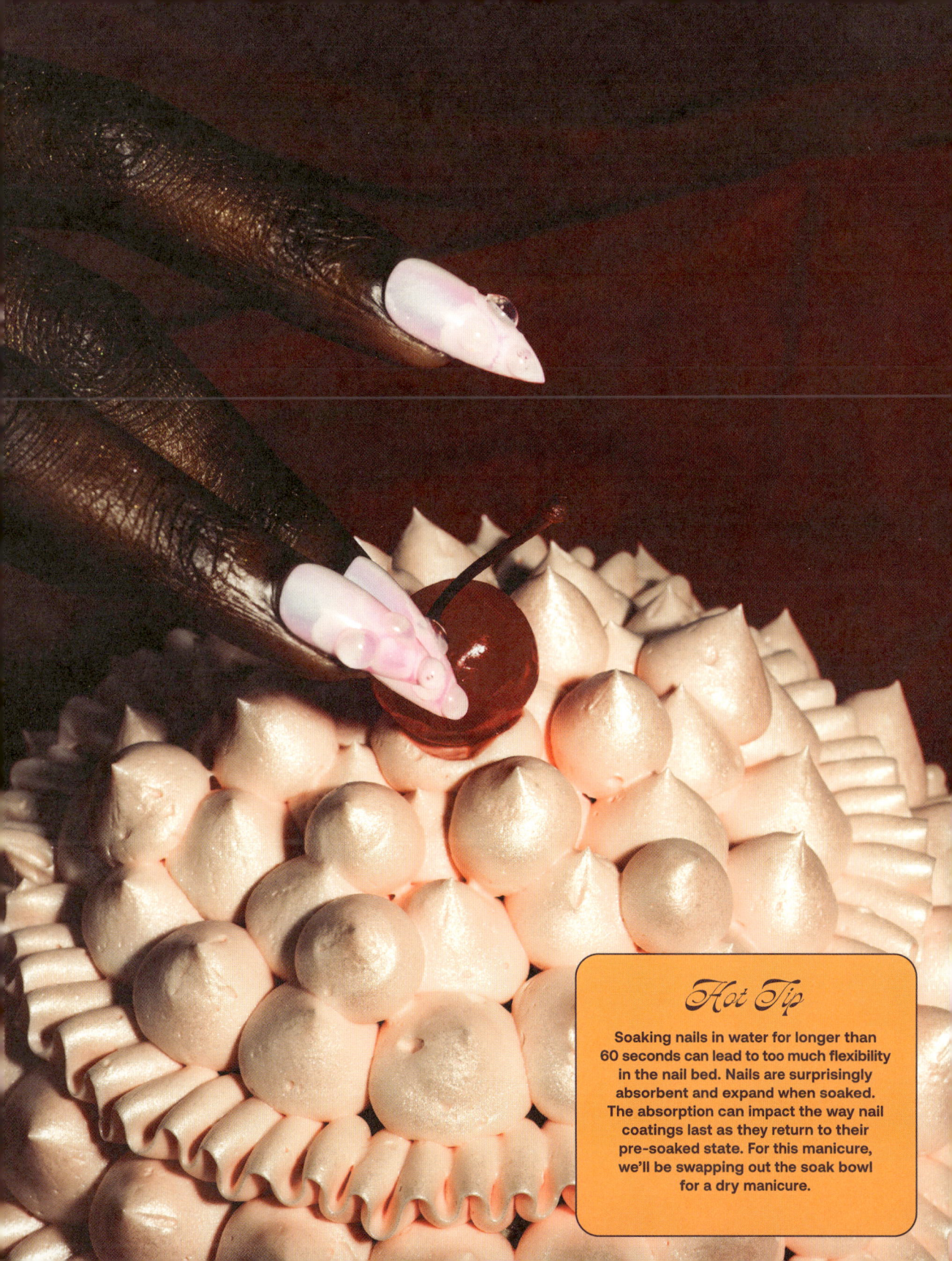

Hot Tip

Soaking nails in water for longer than 60 seconds can lead to too much flexibility in the nail bed. Nails are surprisingly absorbent and expand when soaked. The absorption can impact the way nail coatings last as they return to their pre-soaked state. For this manicure, we'll be swapping out the soak bowl for a dry manicure.

A STEP-BY-STEP
MANICURE

✦

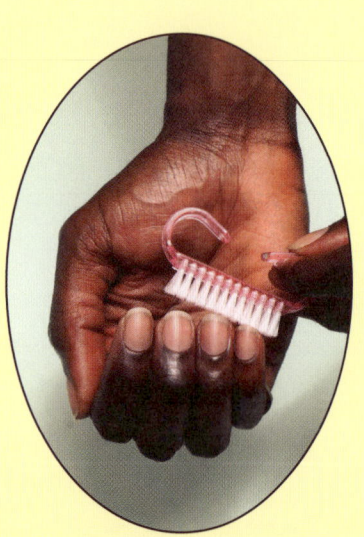 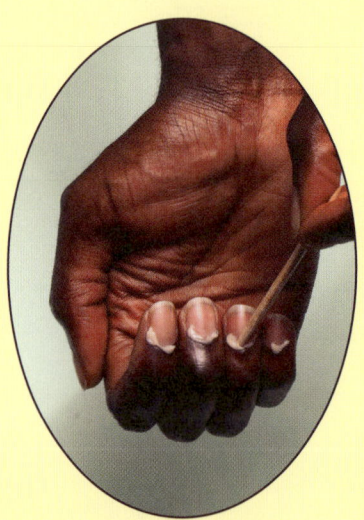 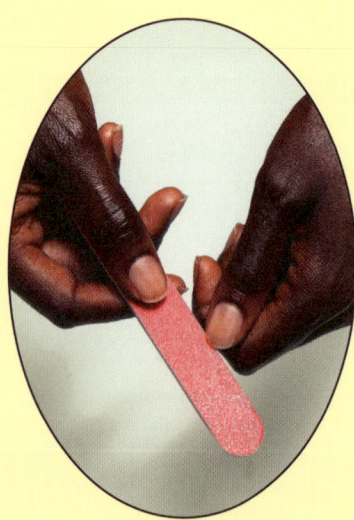

① Wash your hands thoroughly and clean under the fingernails using a nail brush or scratch against your palm while your hands are soapy to release any dirt trapped under your nails.

② Rinse and dry your hands.

③ Apply cuticle remover to the nail bed.

④ Gently push your cuticles back with an orange wood stick or cuticle pusher to remove the sticky cuticle from the nail bed. (While being pushed back and buffed the cuticle will separate from the nail bed and look white in appearance.)

⑤ Wash off the remainder of the cuticle remover.

⑥ Choose your nail shape and file the nail gently to match, being careful to file into the centre of the nail, avoid pressing into the side wall or filing in a sawing motion.

⑦ Without applying pressure, buff across the nail with a fine buffer. Be sure not to miss along the eponychium to ensure the sticky cuticle has lifted from the nail bed.

Mannequin Hands

Make your own cuticle oil

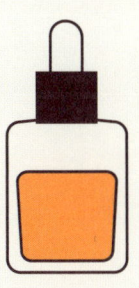

What's all the fuss with cuticle oil? Well, the benefits include preventing dry, cracking skin around the nail, prolonging the life of nail enhancements and maintaining health of the nail.

Let's look at a concoction you can make at home to make sure your hands stay lathered. Play around with what you have, my absolute go-to mix is jojoba and vitamin E oil.

SOME OF MY FAVOURITE OILS TO USE INCLUDE

Jojoba oil
Vitamin E oil
Sunflower oil
Argan oil
Apricot oil
Hempseed oil
Shea oil
Sweet almond oil
Olive oil

You can also add some scented oil to the mix to make the application even more fun. It's also a handy handbag staple for moments when you've forgotten perfume! Be sure to mix any scents in at the recommended percentage and be sure the scent is body safe! If it's not mentioned on the label, best to steer clear.

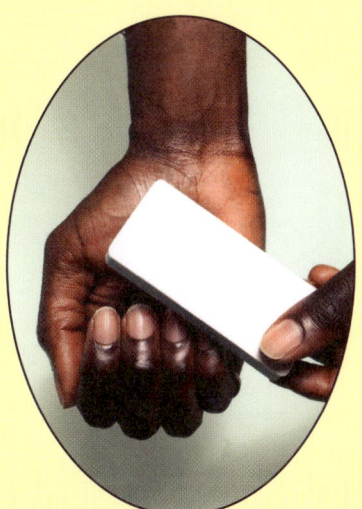
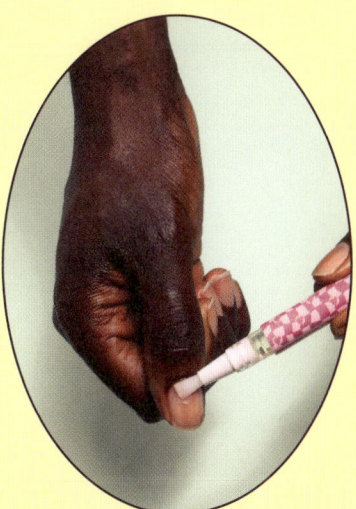

⑧ Spray your fingers with a touch of water and use a super fine buffer to buff away any hardened skin around the nail.

⑨ Carefully trim any hang nails or loose skin but do NOT cut the eponychium.

⑩ Buff with a polishing buffer to achieve a perfect shine across the nail.

⑪ Oil your cuticles generously.

Hot Tip

If you intend on adding a nail coating to the nail, stop your manicure at step 9 and after buffing away any callous skin, wipe your nail with isopropyl alcohol or a chosen nail prep and apply your nail coating of choice. Always finish off with cuticle oil!

FILING

Filing and shaping nails correctly is an art form and takes more time and precision than you'd think. Pause and look at your nails straight out in front of you and then curled in the other way to ensure you're working towards your desired shape as you file.

If you're removing length from the nail hold your file flat across the nail and file until the desired longest point of the nail has been achieved. The file should only move from the outer corners inwards, never sawing back and forth, this creates weakened nails and applies too much pressure to the nail bed. To create the shape, you need to address the corners. Depending on your desired shape this is where the tapering happens. Take the filing one stroke at a time, rushing here is a sure-fire way to file into the side walls. To shape along the sides, ensure your file is sat on an angle under the free edge. Only taper from the corners of the free edge, attempting to 'slim' down the appearance of the nail by filing into the nail bed will cause damage to the side wall.

When shaping from the corners, keep the angle of your file in a position that ensures you don't lose sight of where you're filing.

If you've removed a bit of free edge, there may be fraying under the nail. Use a fine buffer and slide it gently along the underside of the free edge to 'seal' the edge.

When it comes to filing, if you have naturally long nail beds, you'll have noticed the hyponychium, don't push or cut the hyponychium as it can lead to pain and infection.

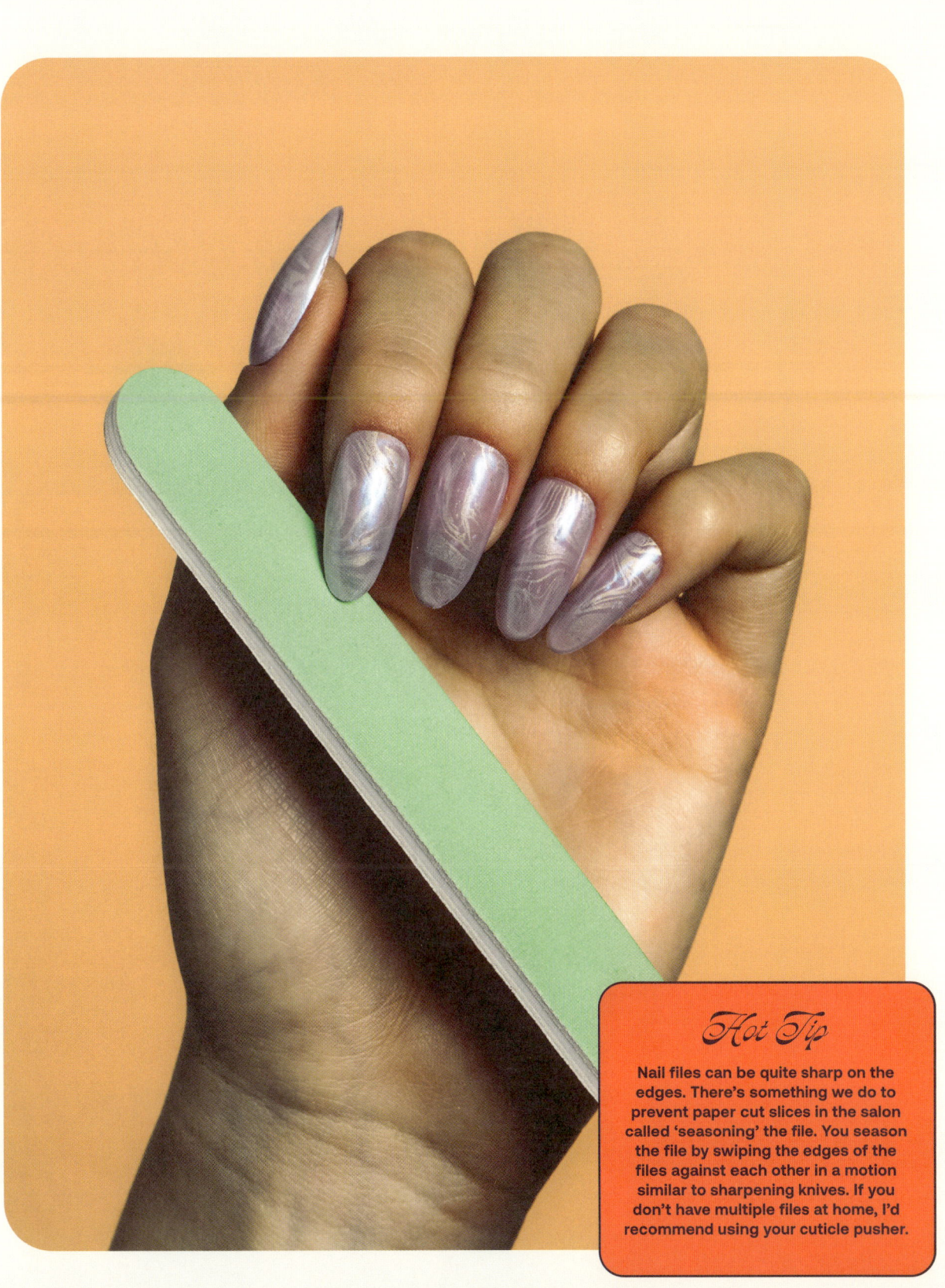

Hot Tip

Nail files can be quite sharp on the edges. There's something we do to prevent paper cut slices in the salon called 'seasoning' the file. You season the file by swiping the edges of the files against each other in a motion similar to sharpening knives. If you don't have multiple files at home, I'd recommend using your cuticle pusher.

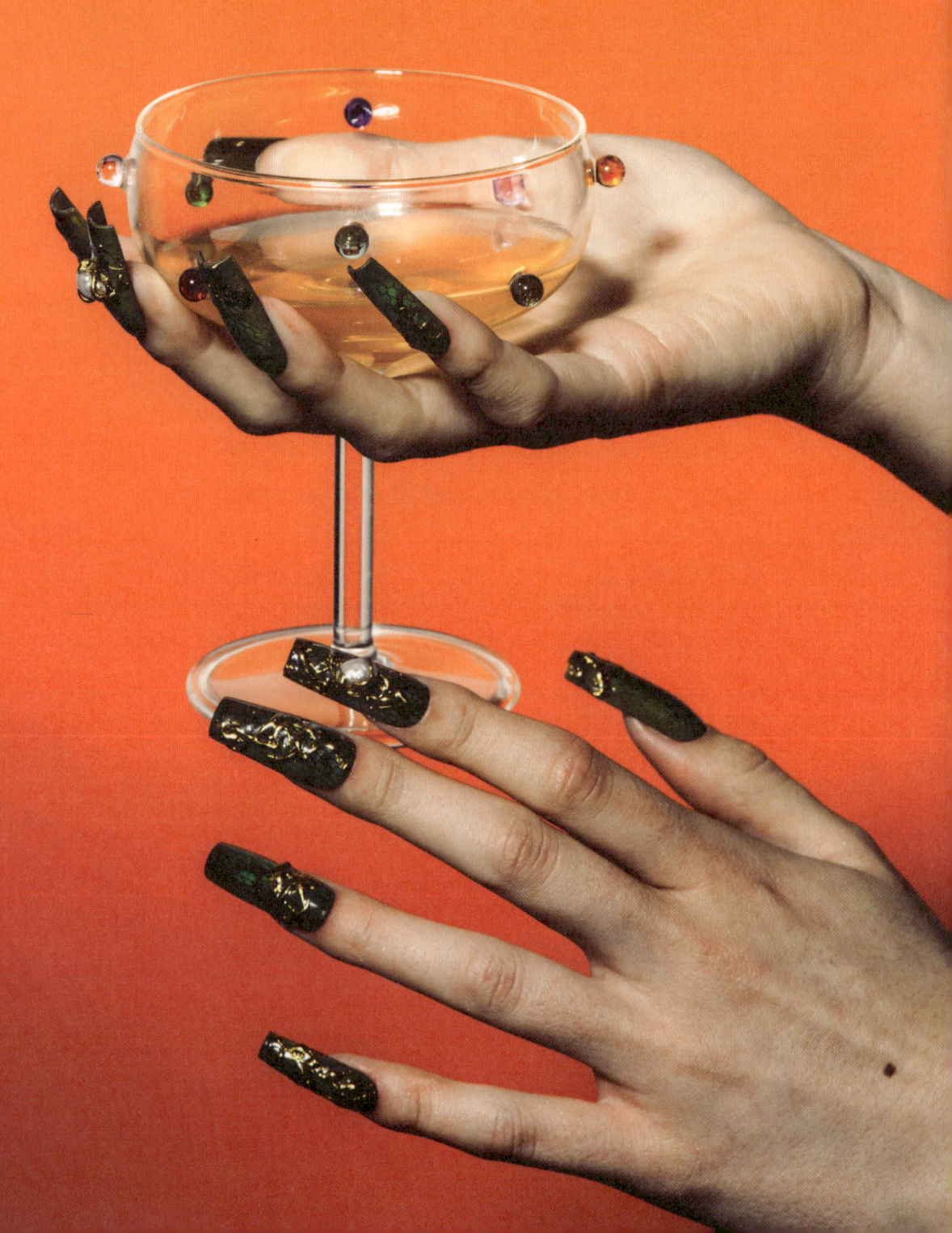

DIY *Nail Art* LOOKS

Whether you're getting ready for an event or pouring yourself a tea and staying in for some TLC, here are 13 designs I've created just for you so you can try your hand at decorating your own nails.

These looks all vary in difficulty and complexity so there's something for everyone!

These designs were chosen to ensure you can create these looks in the comfort of your own home, fittingly because that's where I learnt to do mine. I wanted to make sure that these looks could be built upon and the techniques you'll learn can be mixed and matched to create the set of your dreams. I'm going to run you through how to best utilise different beauty products to create some of the most requested looks from my clients.

Nail art is a lot about trial and error so get ready to play and make these looks your own. Switch out colours to your personal favourites and remember, it isn't permanent, try something new once in a while!

With all that in mind, prepare for the most satisfying feeling of all, getting to say 'I did them!' when someone asks about your nails. So, turn the page and get into the tips and tricks to make you the master of your own set.

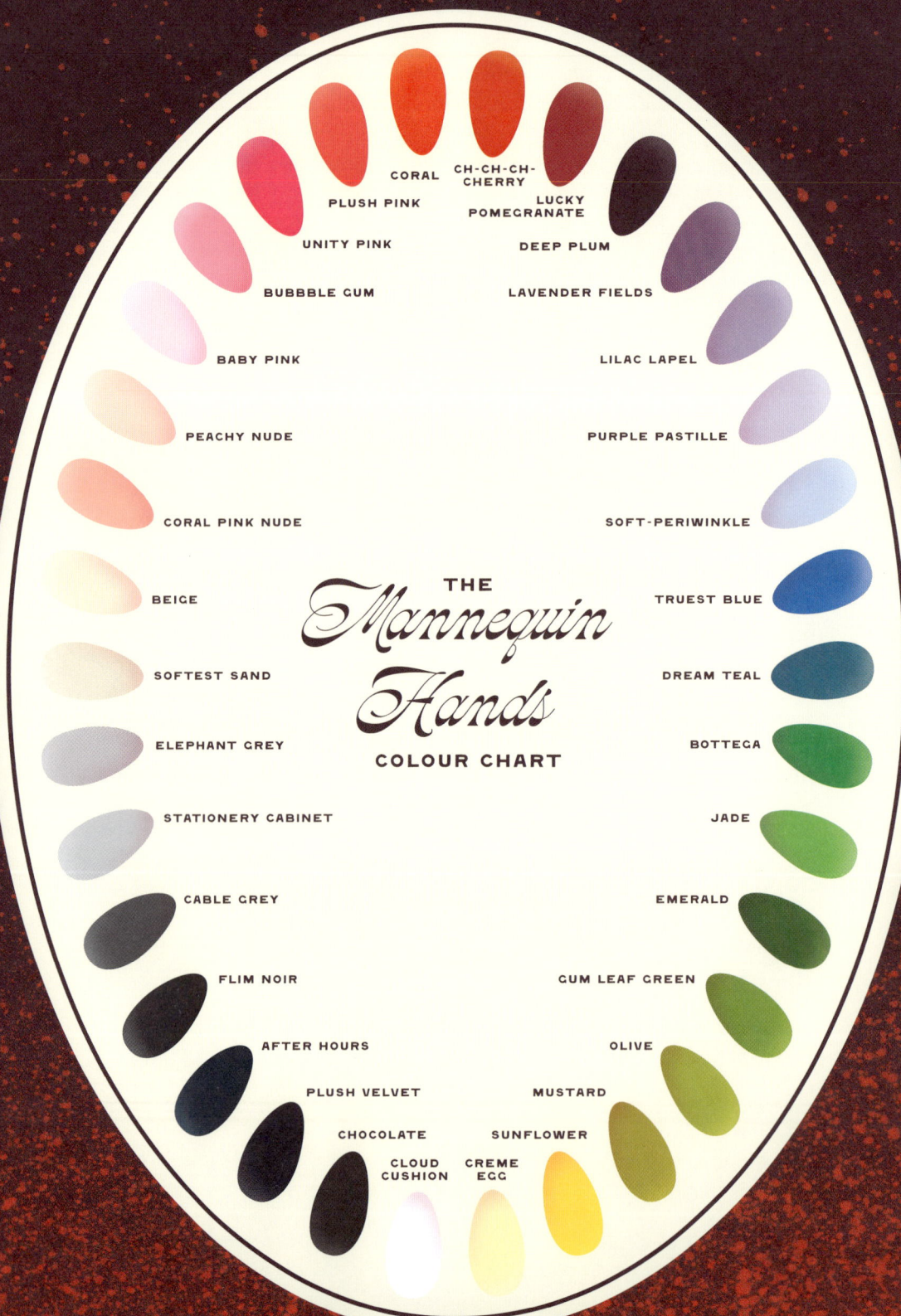

TOOLS KEY

Here's a visual list of all the tools used in the following step-by-step tutorials. At the beginning of each manicure you'll see all the tools needed so you can have everything within arm's reach before starting.

Coats

There are three types of coats used in these tutorials. Base coats are always done first to ensure a smooth colour application. Colour polish is what we'll use for all the sets and designs. Top coats come in both shiny and matte finishes, they seal the design for longer wear.

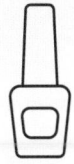 **COLOURS OF YOUR CHOICE**

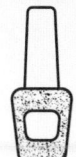 **GLITTER POLISH**

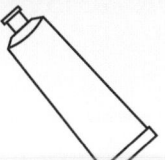 **COLOURED ACRYLIC PAINT**

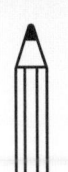 **MARKER**

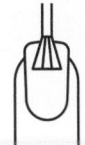 **BASE COAT**

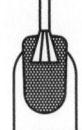 **MATTE COAT**

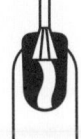 **TOP COAT**

Brushes

All these brushes have a different and specific effect when used in these designs. You can find most of these at your local art or beauty supply store.

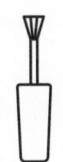 **NAIL BRUSH**

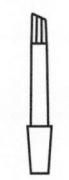 **ANGLED NAIL BRUSH**

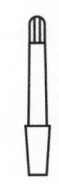 **ROUND NAIL BRUSH**

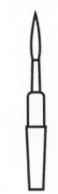 **FINE NAIL ART BRUSH**

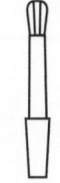 **EYESHADOW BRUSH**

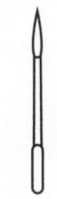 **FINE LINER BRUSH**

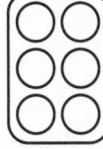 **PALETTE**

This can be anything from a metal make-up artists palette to a post-it note block, my personal favourite!

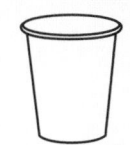 **DISPOSABLE CUP**

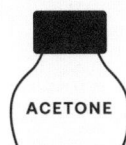 **ACETONE OR NAIL POLISH REMOVER**

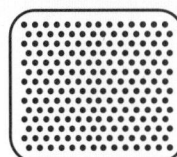 **ACETONE-SOAKED LINT-FREE WIPE**

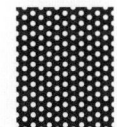 **NON STRETCH MESH**

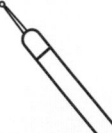 **DOTTING TOOL**

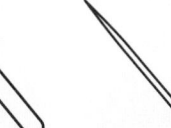 **TOOTH PICK**

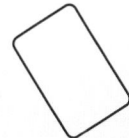 **SCRAPER**

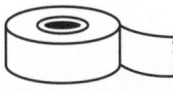 **STICKY TAPE**

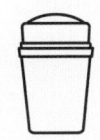 **NAIL STAMPER**

The softer and more flexible the nail stamp, the deeper your French will go. If you have long nails, be sure to use a flexible stamp so it can accommodate the length of your nail.

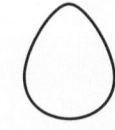 **BEAUTY OR EYE-SHADOW SPONGE**

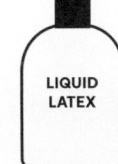 **LIQUID LATEX**

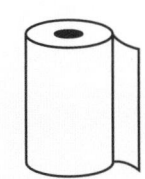 **PAPER TOWELS**

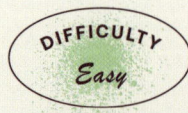 DIFFICULTY Easy

Gradient nails

TIME
15 MIN

+

Just like the French tip, gradient nails can be executed through a couple of methods. With a clear or nude base, French tips and gradient nails alike both have minimal visual grow out making them a staple for busy nail art lovers, or those who hate to see that grown out gap. There are all kinds of gradients but for Method 1 let's start with the easiest.

WHAT YOU'LL NEED

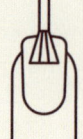 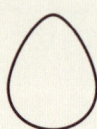 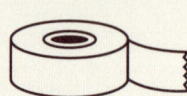 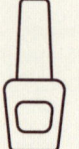 × 2+

METHOD 1

① Apply your base coat.

② Tap the beauty sponge on the sticky side of the tape to ensure your nail look isn't ruined by dust and fluff.

③ Tap a beauty sponge into your chosen colour. Careful not to tap more than a couple of times as the polish is drying to avoid creating unwanted texture.

④ Press the polish-soaked beauty sponge onto the tip of the nail.

⑤ Repeat step 3 moving further and further up to the tip of the nail for even coverage and a smooth gradient. Repeat steps 4 and 5 in as many graduating colours as you like.

⑥ Once dry apply your top coat.

Hot Tip

The smoothest gradients are achieved with a little colour theory, to achieve a super seamless gradient the colour furthest from the tip should be closest to the base colour of your nail bed. Of course, there are no rules so if you're going for mass contrast blend on with a wild and playful colour!

CONTINUED ☞

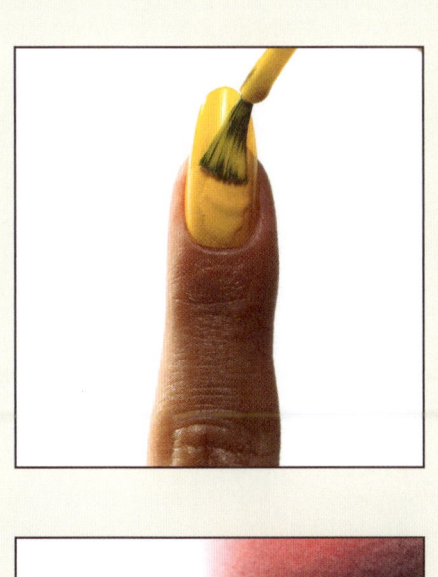
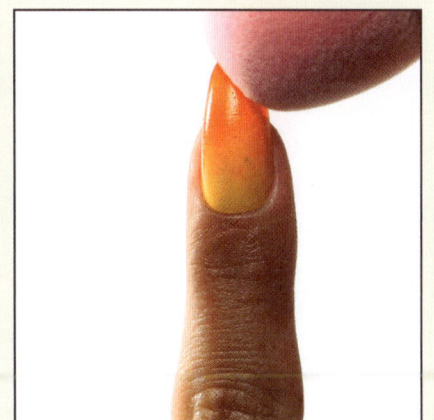
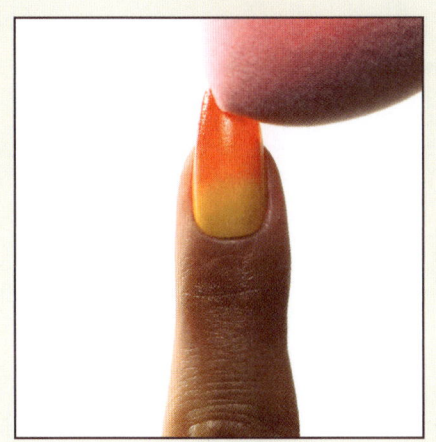
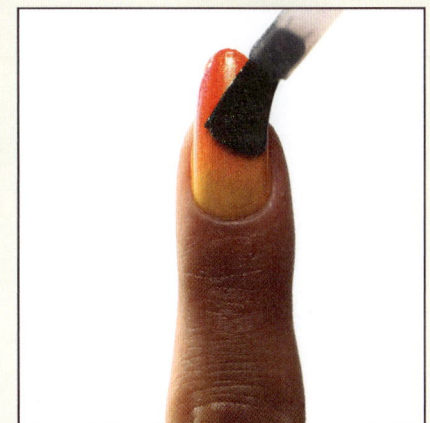
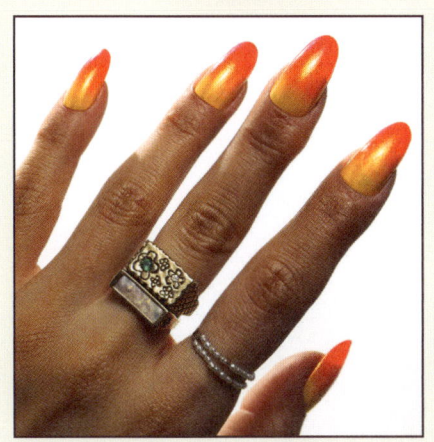
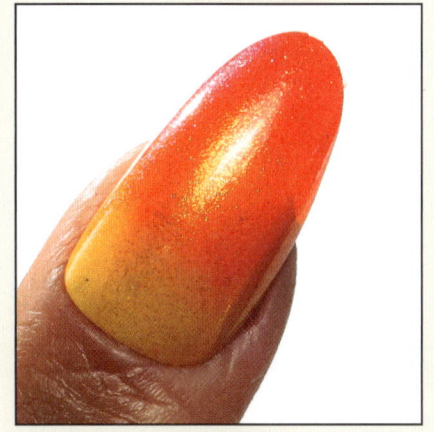

Hands-on Tutorials

(CONTINUED 👉)

Method 1 wasn't your favourite? Not to worry, pull out a glitter polish and let's try something a little different, meet Method 2.

WHAT YOU'LL NEED

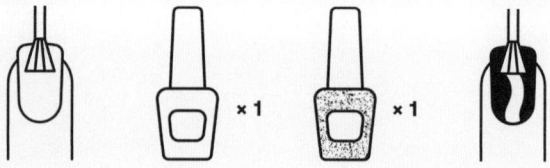

METHOD 2

① Apply your base coat.

② Apply your base colour.

③ Gently swipe off as much glitter from the brush as possible before lightly painting the nail three quarters of the way down the nail.

④ Repeat step 3 only coating half of the nail.

⑤ Repeat step 3 this time only coating one quarter of the nail.

⑥ Once dry apply your top coat.

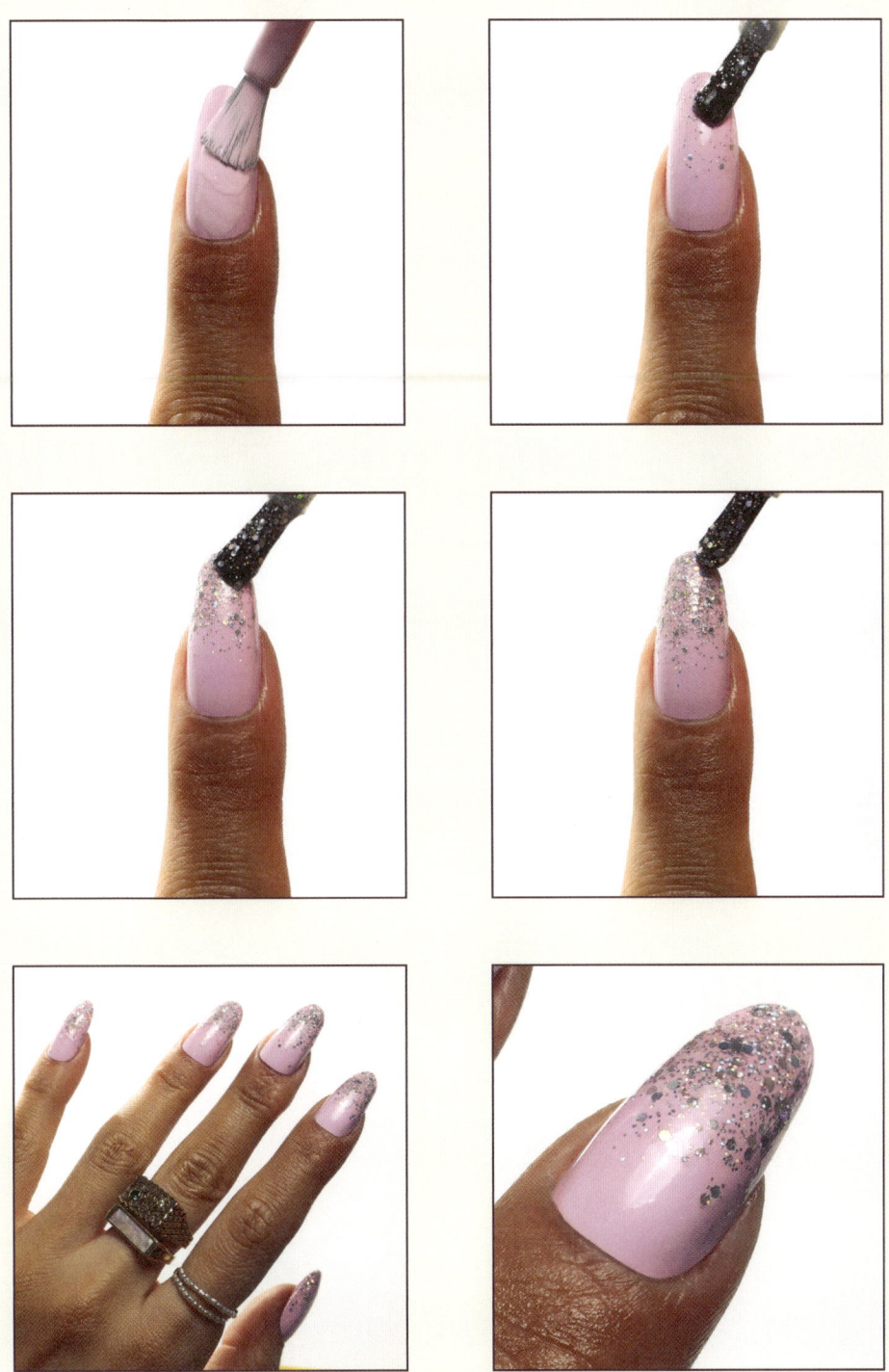

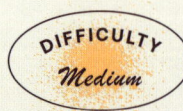

French tips

TIME
20 MIN

+

They're a classic, an homage to the natural nail, the French tip could be considered the origin story of nail art as it stands yet getting it perfect is tough. Let's look at a few tips and tricks to make a French tip as easy to do as it looks.

WHAT YOU'LL NEED

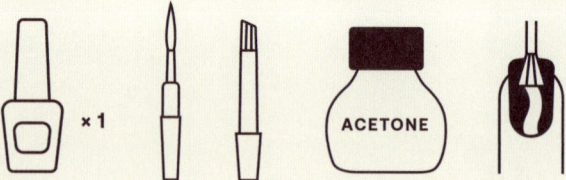

METHOD 1

① Swipe the chosen colour for your tip across the top of your nail, if you'd like the tip to mimic the natural smile line ensure the 'white' of your natural nail is covered in the polish. Don't use too much product, it'll create a mess, and your clean base will be marbled with the tip colour once you apply your top coat.

② Dip a nail art brush, my preference is an angled brush, into the acetone.

③ Swipe the brush across the nail from the deepest point of the French tip from one side to the other.

④ Repeat step 3 until you have a clean smile line.

⑤ Once dry apply your top coat.

CONTINUED ☞

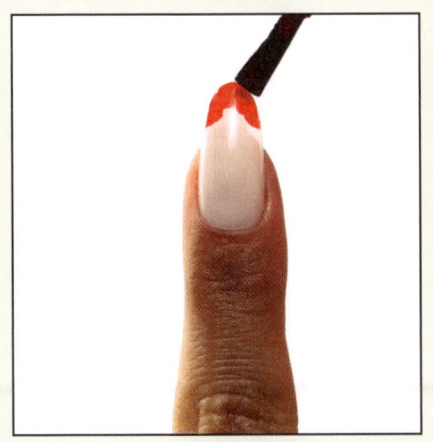
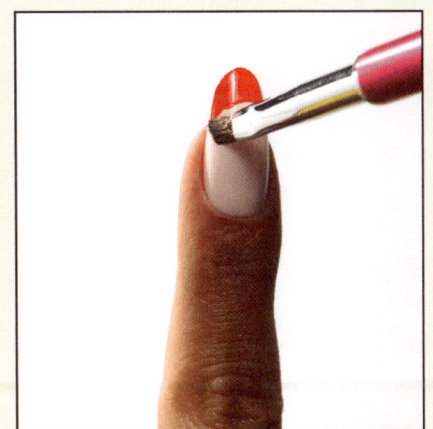
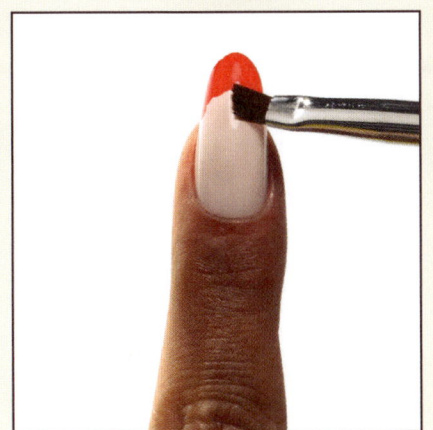
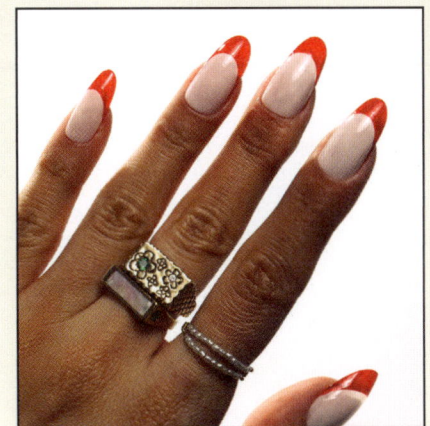
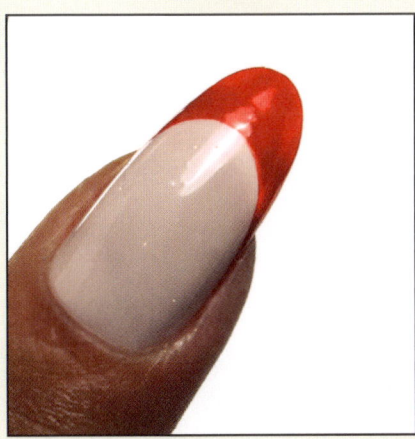

Hands-on Tutorials

(CONTINUED ☞)

Ok, so you're a little too heavy handed and acetone happy for Method 1?
Let's try another approach.

WHAT YOU'LL NEED

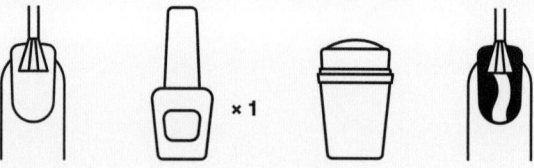

METHOD 2

① Apply your base coat.

② Swipe the chosen colour for your tip across a nail stamp.

③ Firmly and slowly press the tip of your nail into the polish on the stamp.

④ While maintaining the position of the stamp at a 90-degree angle, tilt to the left and right to ensure the French tip is elongated along the side wall of the nails.

⑤ Once dry apply your top coat.

(CONTINUED ☞)

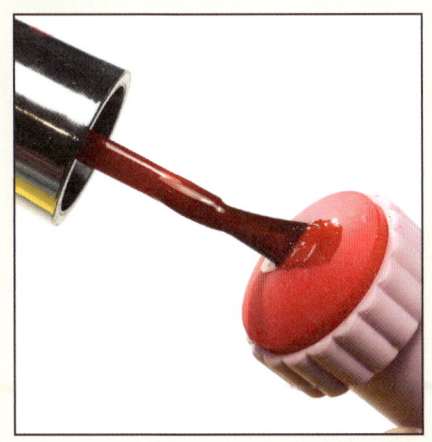
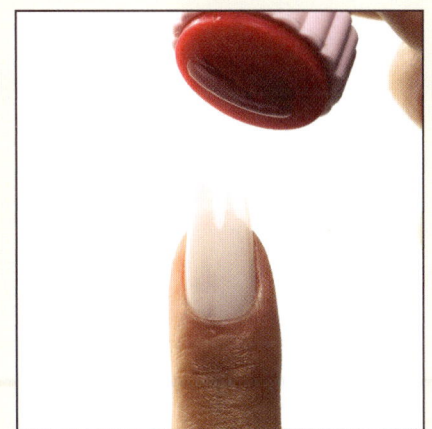
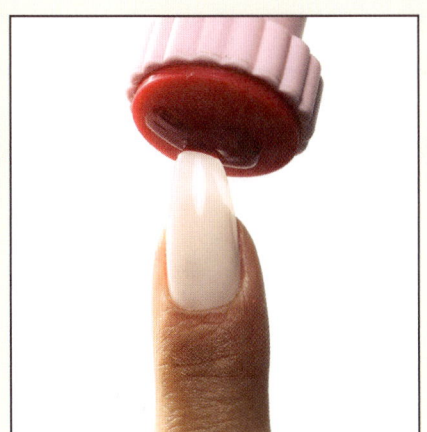
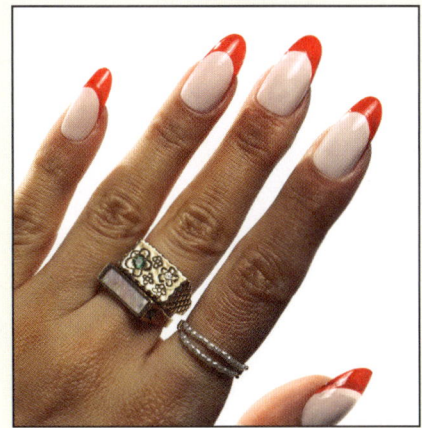
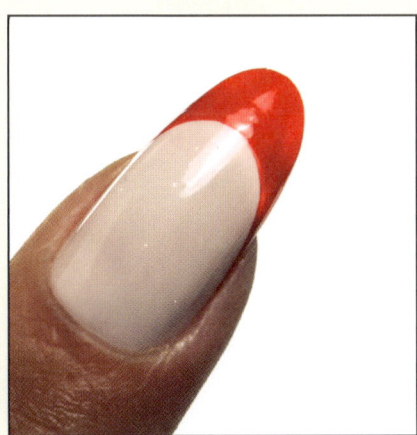

Hands-on Tutorials

CONTINUED 👉

Method 2 requires a nail stamp and the one you bought is 7-10 business days away? Alright, let's try another option.

WHAT YOU'LL NEED

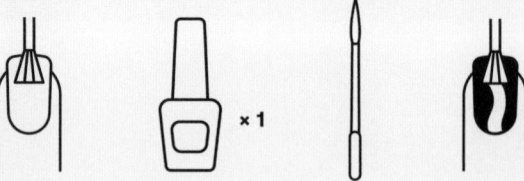

METHOD 3

① Apply your base coat.

② Dip your fine liner brush into your chosen colour and swipe from left to the centre.

③ Repeat step 2 but this time swipe from right to the centre. If the polish is beginning to thicken on your liner brush, swipe the brush between a lint-free wipe coated in acetone.

④ Fill in the bare space between the smile line and the tip.

⑤ Once dry apply your top coat.

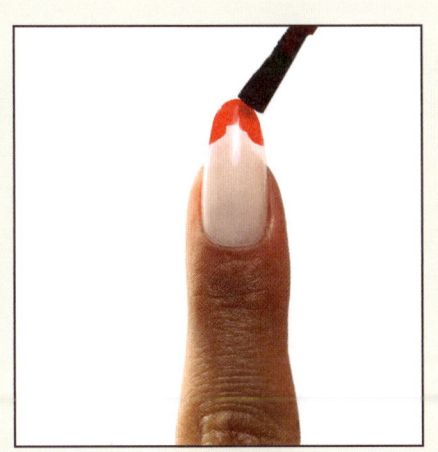
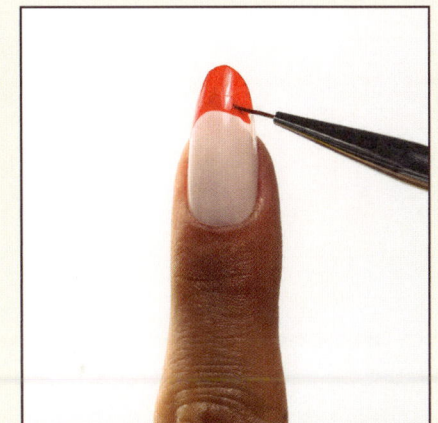
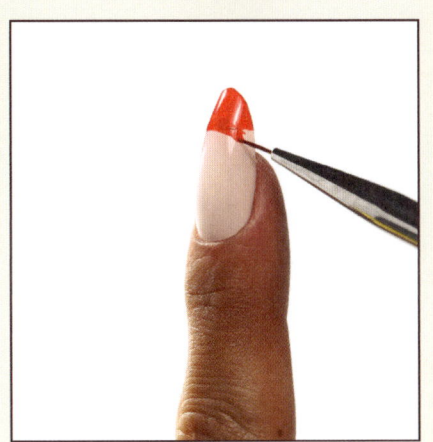
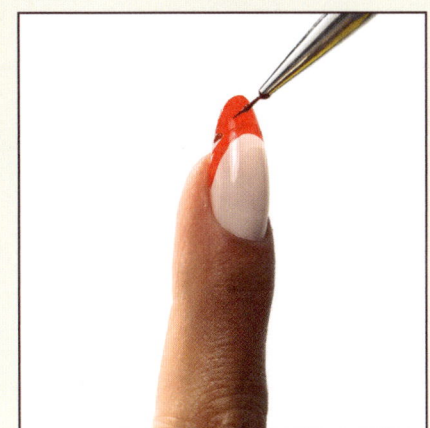
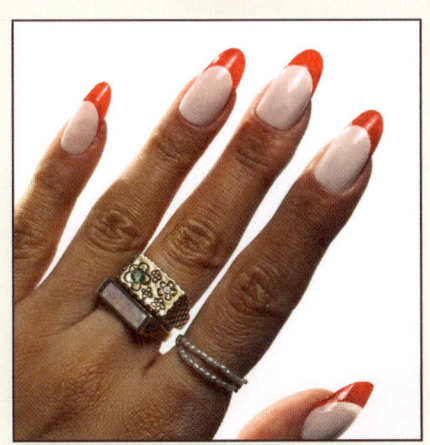
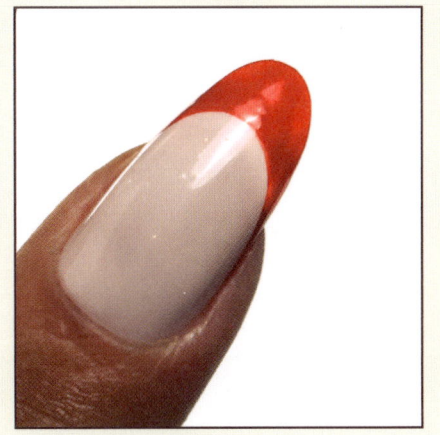

Hands-on Tutorials

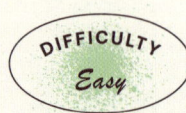

Snakeskin nails

TIME: 15 MIN

I love a snakeskin look more than anything, they can be channelled in any colours and they pop!

WHAT YOU'LL NEED

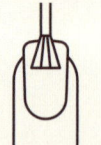 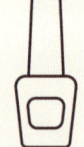 ×3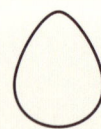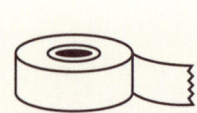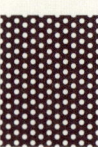

METHOD

① Apply your base coat.

② Apply your base colour.

③ Stamp your sponge on the sticky side of the tape – this ensures your look will remain dust and fluff free!

④ Dab the sponge in your first colour and tap the sponge on your palette a couple of times to ensure the colour is distributed evenly.

⑤ Hold the mesh taut over your finger, edge to edge is best to ensure the mesh doesn't move.

⑥ Tap the sponge over the mesh to cover the nail evenly. Don't move the mesh just yet!

⑦ To add a little extra dimension, go in with a slightly lighter colour and tap the colour in a line down the middle of the nail.

⑧ Peel your mesh away to reveal the pattern.

⑨ Once dry apply your top coat.

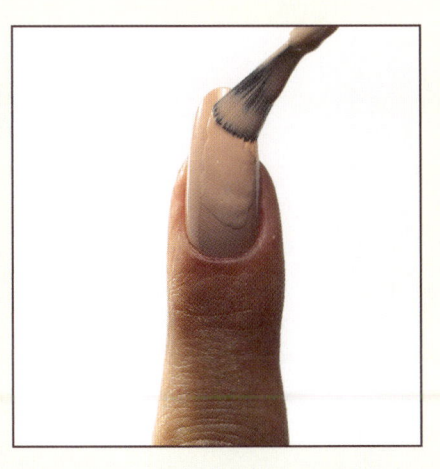
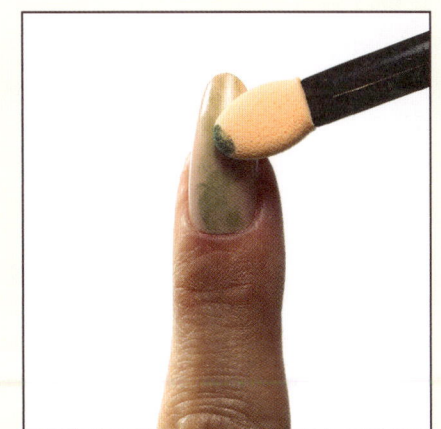
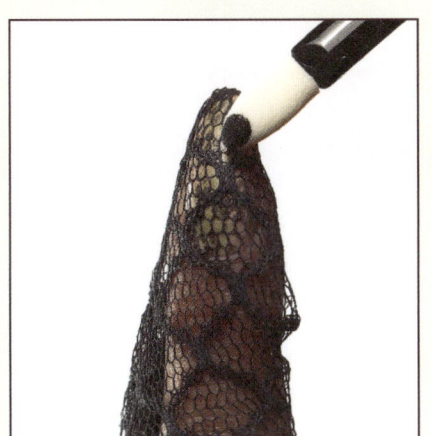
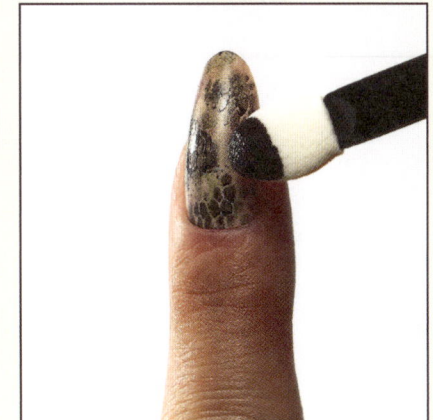
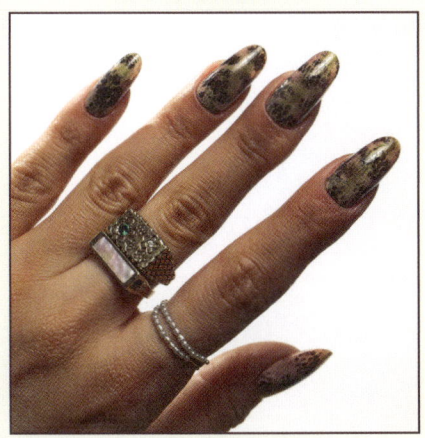
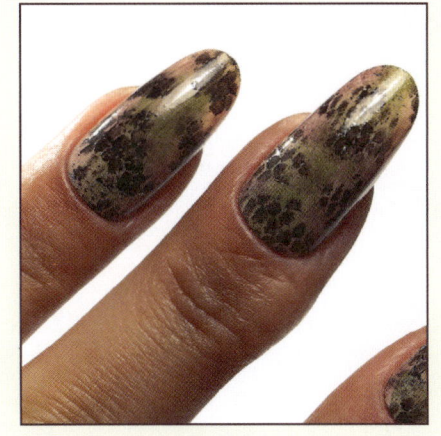

Hands-on Tutorials

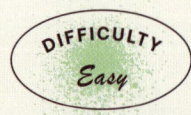 # Leopard print

TIME
15 MIN

+

There's something about a leopard print that never gets old. It can be done in any colours, it can be worn as a full nail or a French tip, but anything that conjures up the glory of Fran Fine or Kylie Minogue's tour looks, makes for a staple in the world of nail art.

WHAT YOU'LL NEED

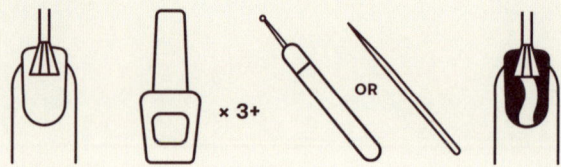

METHOD

① Apply your base coat.

② Apply your base colour.

③ Using a dotting tool or toothpick, apply spaced out imperfect dots.

④ In a darker colour, dot broken marks around your first dots.

⑤ For dimension add a few random imperfect smaller dots by dotting with a super light touch in any large gaps.

⑥ Once dry apply your top coat.

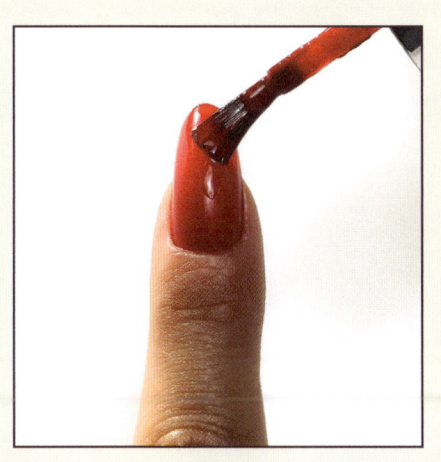
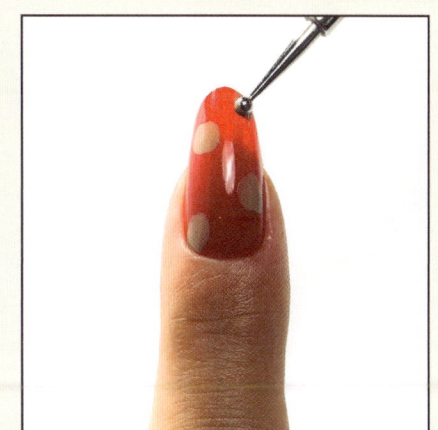
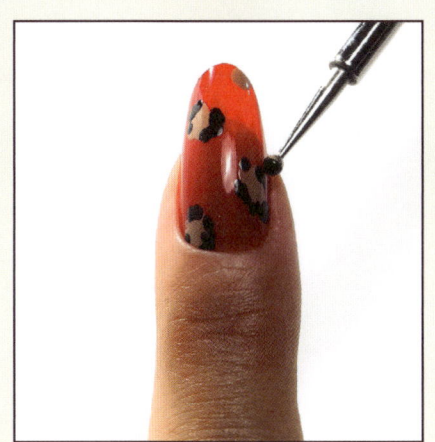
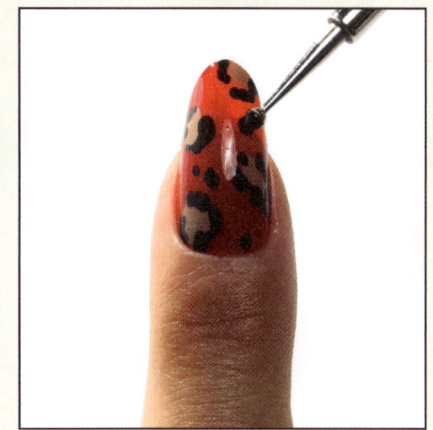
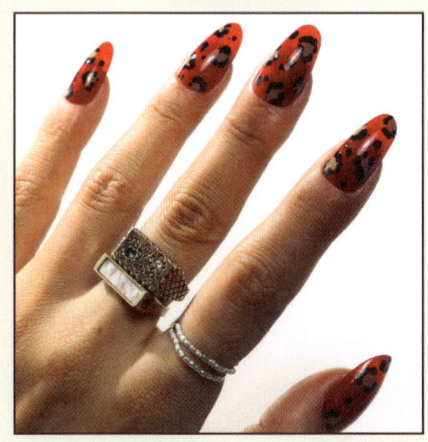
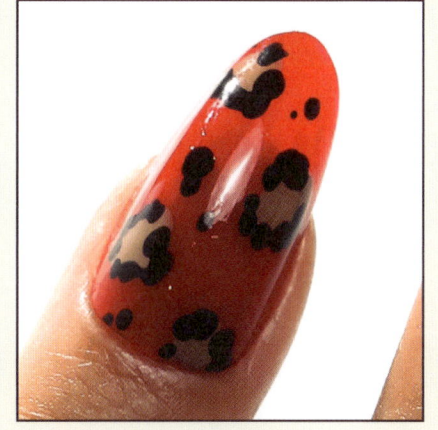

Hands-on Tutorials

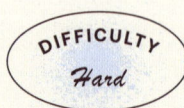 DIFFICULTY Hard

Checkerboard print

TIME
40 MIN

+

They're a real tedious effort but gosh do they look good! Checkerboard print is the perfect base for more art or can be the star of the show. Any colour iteration looks great, but a little extra contrast makes the print pop.

WHAT YOU'LL NEED

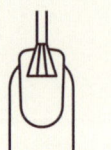 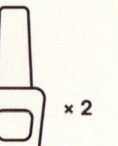 × 2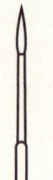

METHOD

① Apply your base coat.

② Apply your base colour.

③ Using a fine liner brush with a colour of your choice create a fine vertical line down the centre of the nail. The more spaced out, the bigger the check, the closer together, the finer the check.

④ Repeat step 3 on either side of the centre line.

⑤ Paint a horizontal line across the centre of the nail.

⑥ Repeat step 5 on either side of the first horizontal line.

⑦ Fill in every second square.

⑧ Once dry apply your top coat.

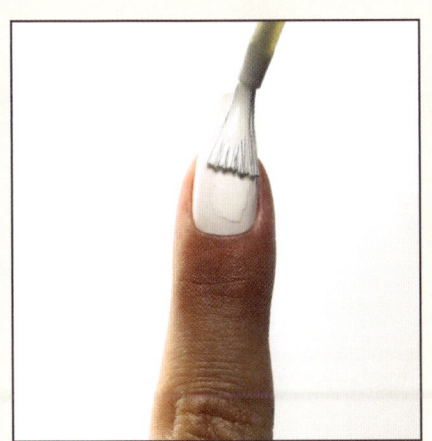 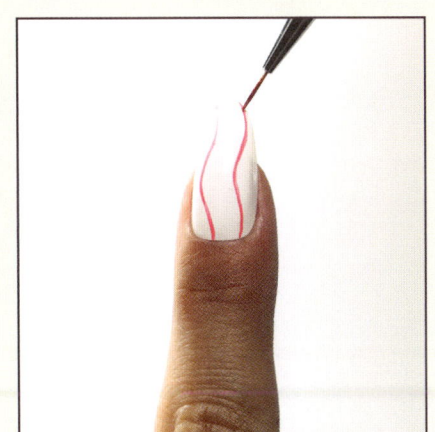

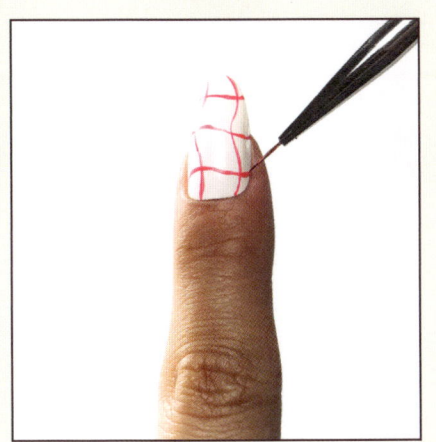 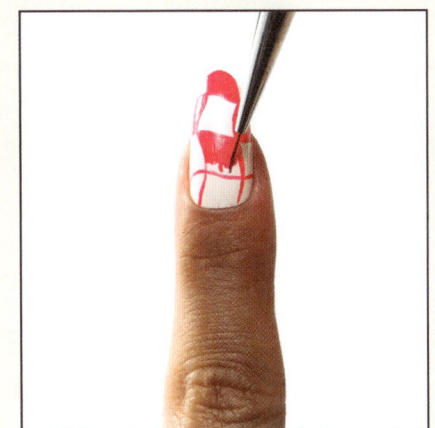

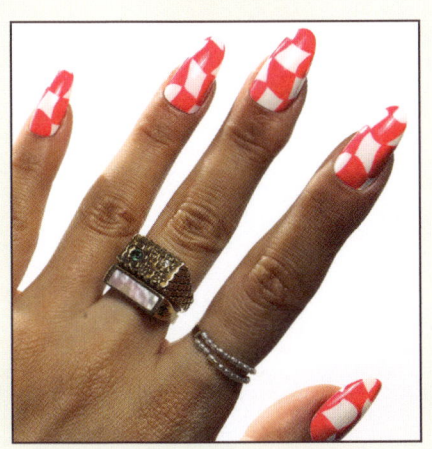 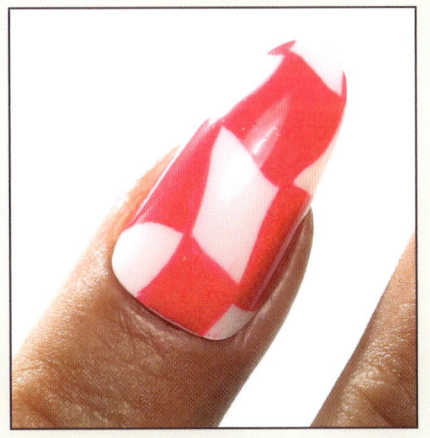

Hands-on Tutorials

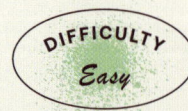

Optical illusion

TIME
20 MIN

It's incredible how something as simple as placing dots in different sizes, shapes and colours can create the look of an optical illusion on the nail. The more contrast, the more dots, the more colour, the better!

WHAT YOU'LL NEED

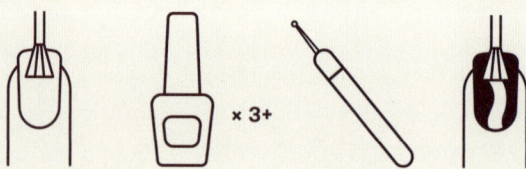

METHOD

① Apply your base coat.

② Apply your base colour.

③ Add a row of dots graduating in size.

④ Once dry, add another row of dots, ideally in a contrasting colour just slightly off the line of the previous dots.

⑤ Repeat step 4 as many times as you please to create a dynamic pattern across the nail.

⑥ Once dry, apply your top coat.

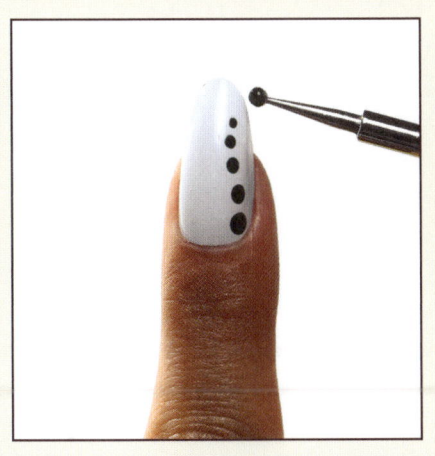
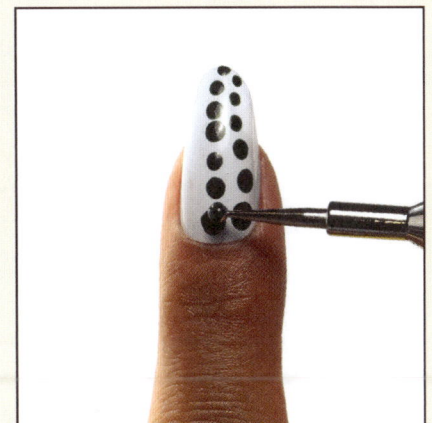
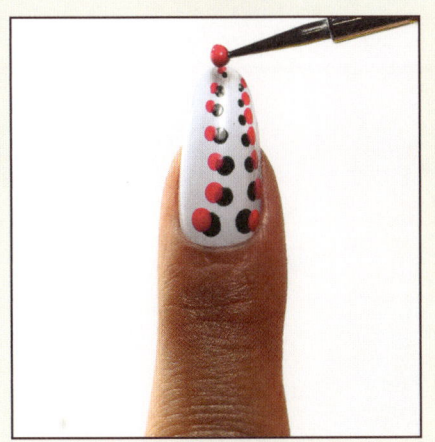
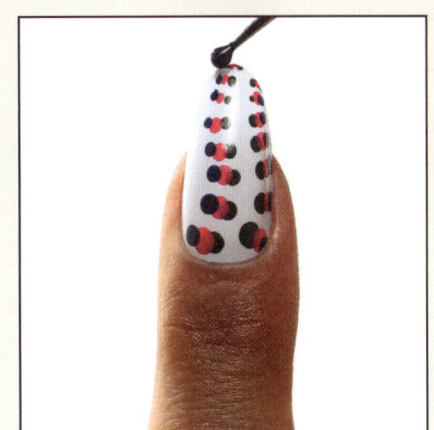
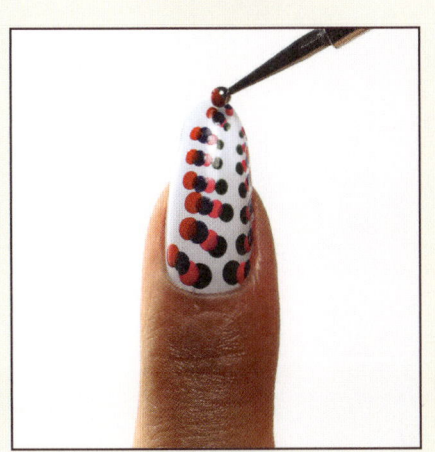
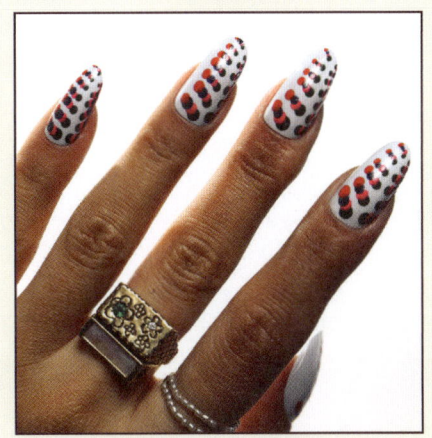

Hands-on Tutorials

Fruit salad

DIFFICULTY *Hard*

TIME 40 MIN

It doesn't matter how cute or classic someone likes their nails, a little fresh produce on a set never fails. I always choose between detailed or cartoon styles and if you want a consistent tip on where your shading or shine line should be, look to the emoji keyboard.

WHAT YOU'LL NEED

 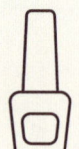 × 3+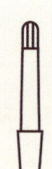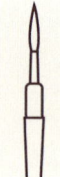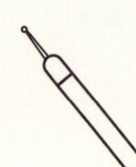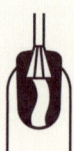

METHOD

① Apply your base coat.

② Apply your base colours or design, for the example in the picture I've gone with some contrasting colours so the fruits pop! For placement of the designs, I like to keep the smaller fruits on the pinkie and save some of the more detailed fruits for the nails with a little more space!

FOR A BANANA

① Take a yellow and create a crescent curve with a round brush.

② Once dry, add a touch of brown for the stem with a fine liner brush.

FOR A WATERMELON

① Start with a pink triangle.

② Frame the lower side of the pink triangle with a light green curve.

③ Repeat step 2 in a darker green slightly further out.

④ Apply black tear drops in the centre of the pink triangle.

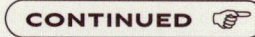

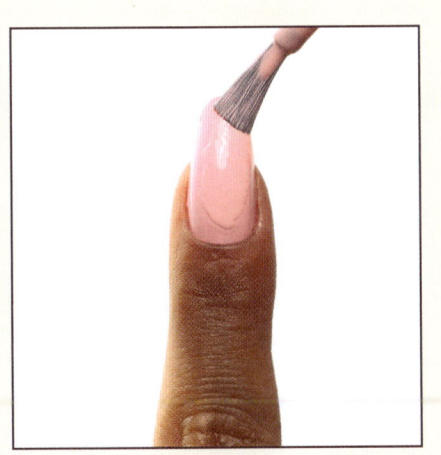
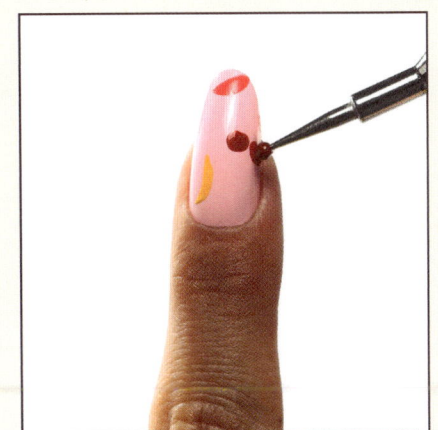
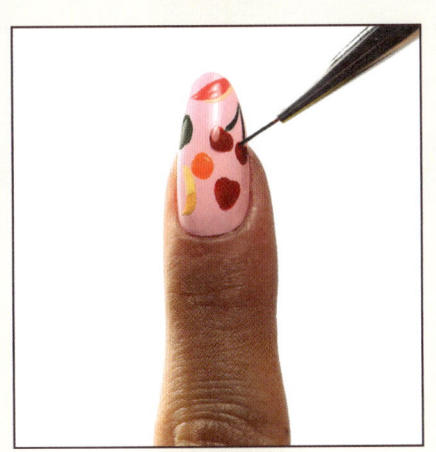
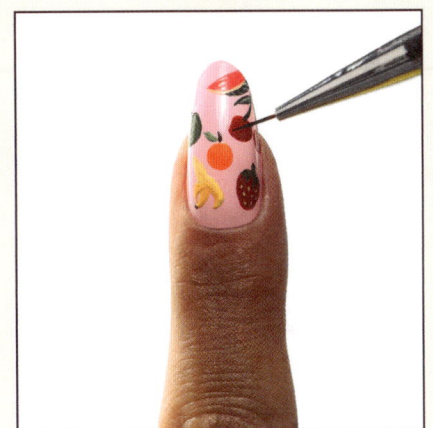
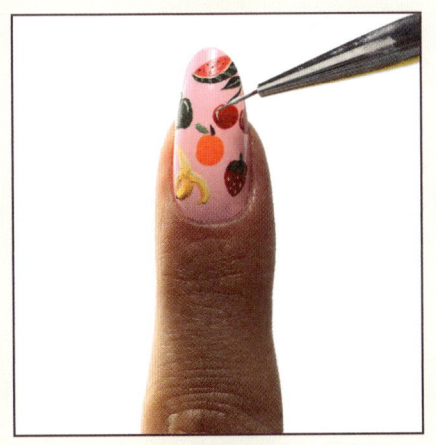
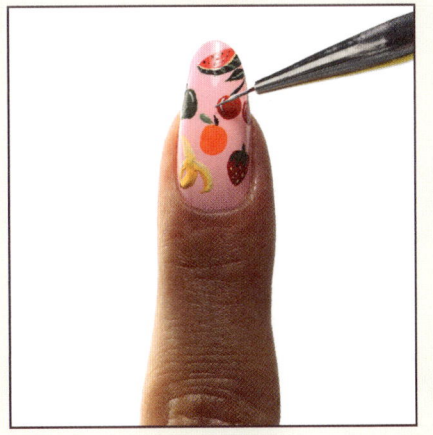

Hands-on Tutorials

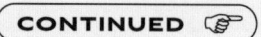

FOR AN APPLE

① Drag out two ovals with a dotting tool.

② Using a fine liner brush add a brown stem.

③ Using a different shade of green, brush a small flick and meet the same shape underneath to form the leaf.

FOR AN ORANGE

① Create a circle with a dotting tool.

② Using a fine liner brush add a brown stem.

③ Using green polish, brush a small flick and meet the same shape underneath to form the leaf.

FOR A STRAWBERRY

① Dot three red spots close together and join them with your dotting tool.

② With a fine liner brush and green polish create an upside-down 'W' on the tip of the red shape and flick a dash of green from where you want the top of the stem to be placed, to the well of the upside-down W for the stem.

FOR CHERRIES

① Apply two red dots close together and drag your dotting tool in a curve between the two to create one cherry. With a little space from the first, repeat for the second cherry.

② With a fine liner brush and a deep green, flick two brush strokes from where you'd like the stems to meet in a curved line above the centre of the two cherries to the cherry tops. Going from the cherry to the stem ensures the line goes from thick to thin.

③ Where the two green lines meet, add a brown stem.

TO FINISH

① Once dry apply your top coat.

141

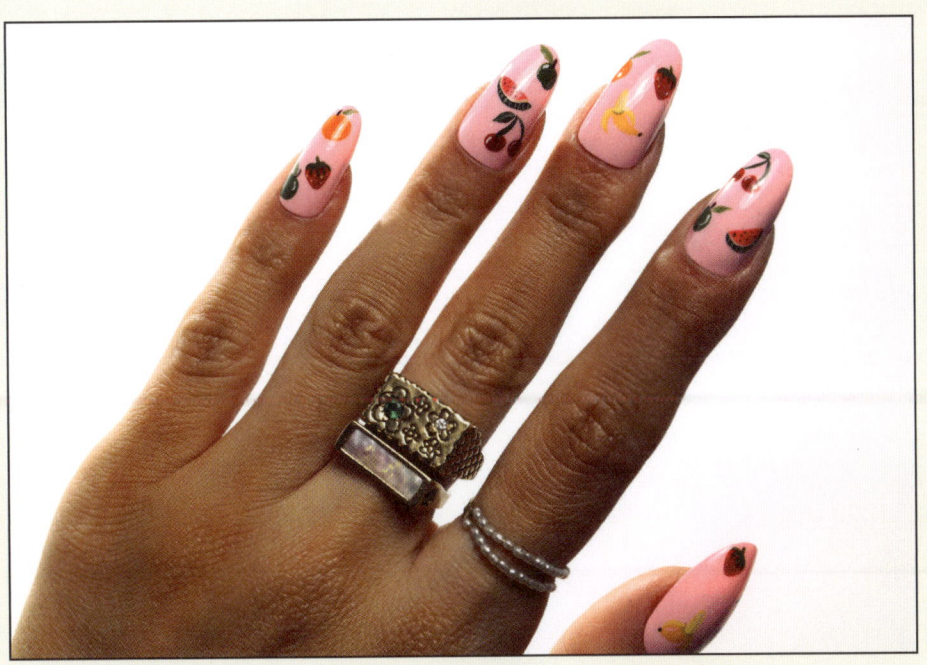

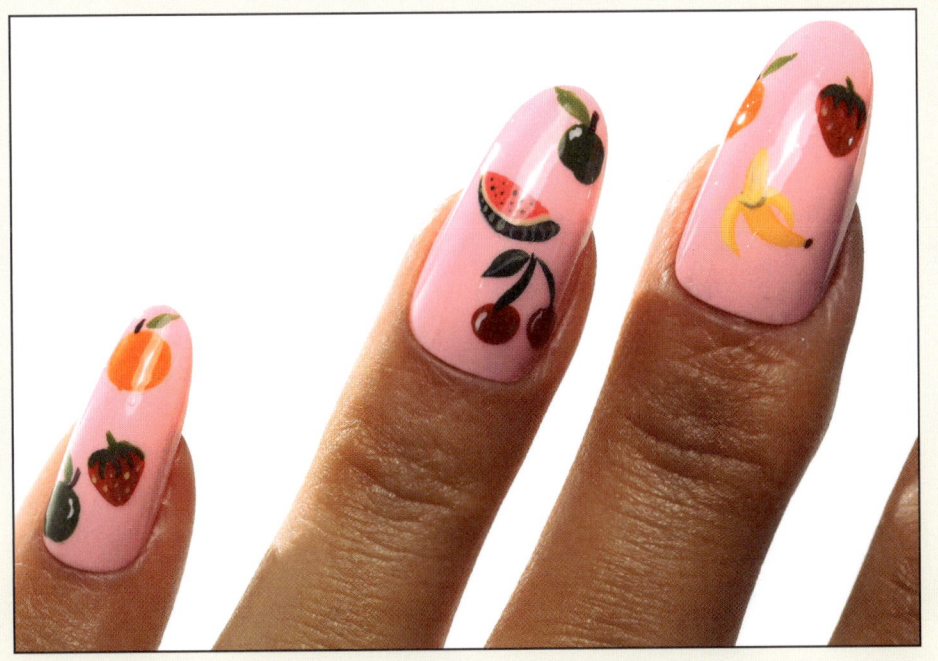

Hands-on Tutorials

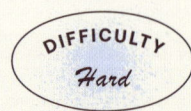

Starry night nails

TIME 40 MIN

Sometimes the wildest looks are the easiest to achieve.
Pull out your old acrylic paints and make Monet fingertips.

WHAT YOU'LL NEED

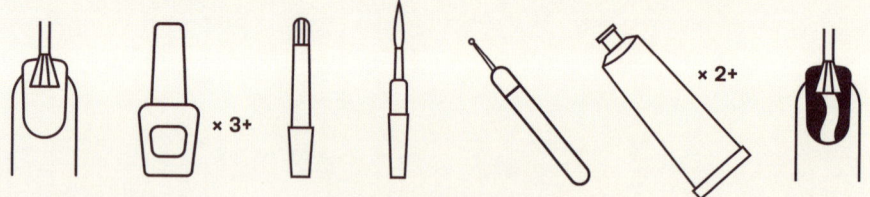

METHOD

① Apply your base coat.

② Apply a deep navy for your base colour.

③ With a round brush and blue acrylic paint, mark out the centre of the design with washy, painterly strokes. If you're feeling confident, pick up a touch of white and a little darker blue to let the paints do some of the detailed shading for you.

④ Apply a teal green just below your centre point, again adding some darker and lighter green to the brush for more detailed shading.

⑤ With a fine brush, add white detailing in the clouds. Then, with a darker colour, add some details to the deepest points in the painting.

⑥ Using yellow, apply circular shapes to create the stars, this can be done with your brush or a dotting tool.

⑦ Once dry apply your top coat.

Mannequin Hands

143

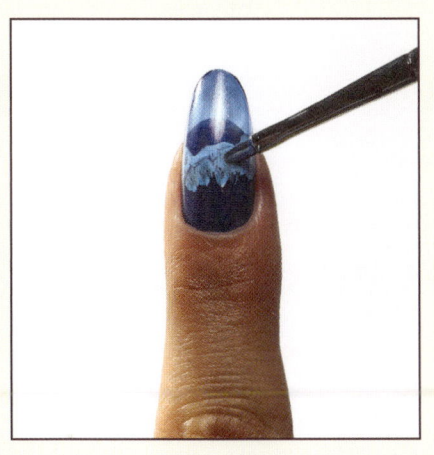
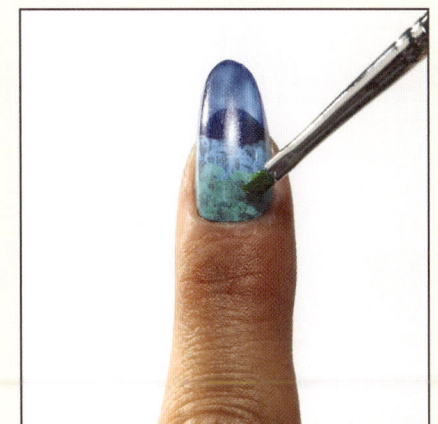
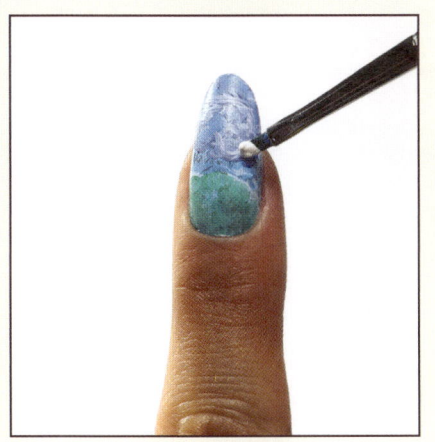
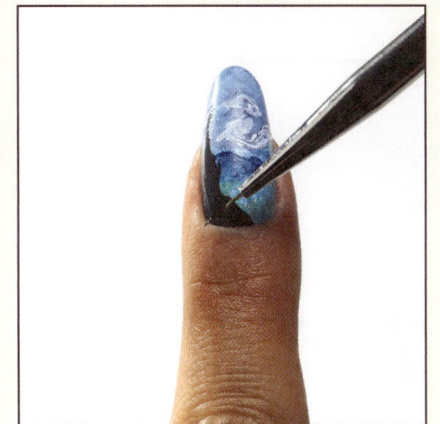
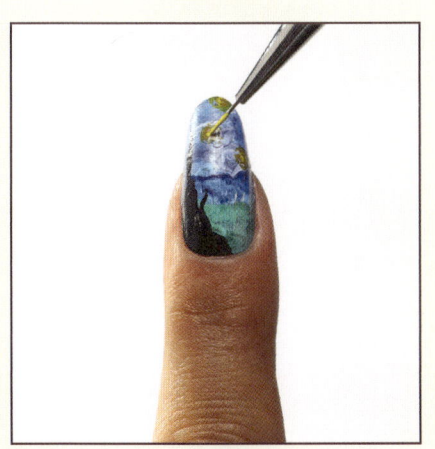
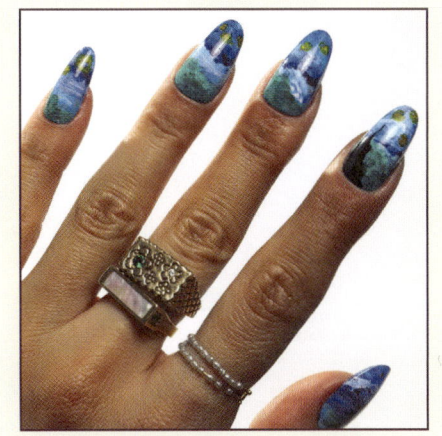

Hands-on Tutorials

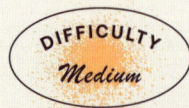

Poison Frog

TIME: 30 MIN

In any colour way, or every colour way across the hands, these are the perfect example of emulating a little nature on the nail.

WHAT YOU'LL NEED

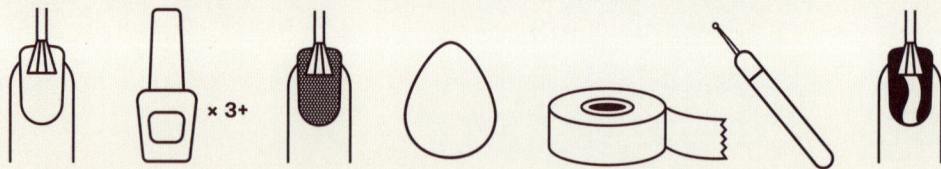

METHOD

① Apply your base coat.

② Apply your base colour.

③ Apply your matte top coat.

④ Tap the beauty sponge on the sticky side of the tape to ensure your nail look isn't ruined by dust and fluff.

⑤ Once your base coat is dry, tap your sponge in another colour and press it down the centre or across the base or tip.

⑥ Using a dotting tool create dragged out shapes and dots in black.

⑦ Repeat step 6 until you're happy with how busy the nail is.

⑧ Once dry apply your top coat.

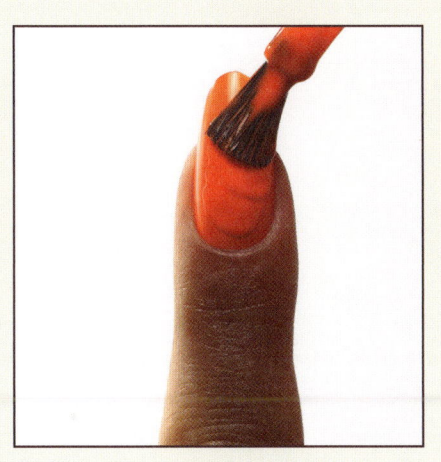
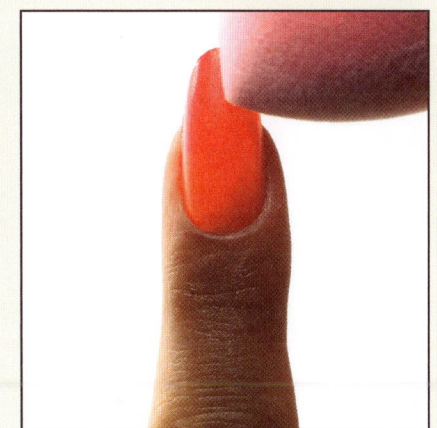
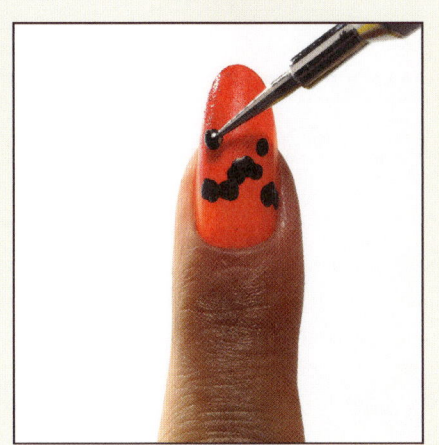
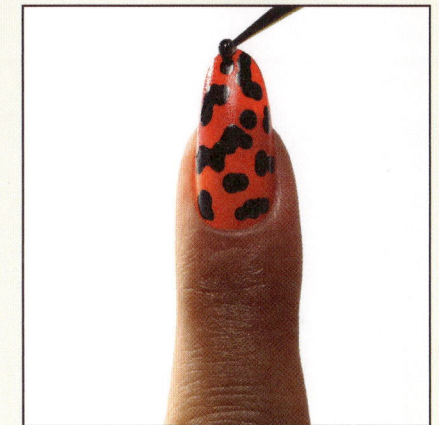
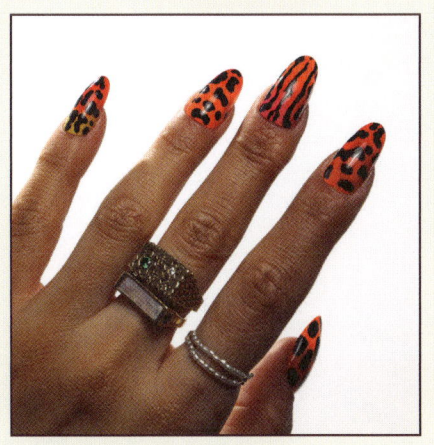
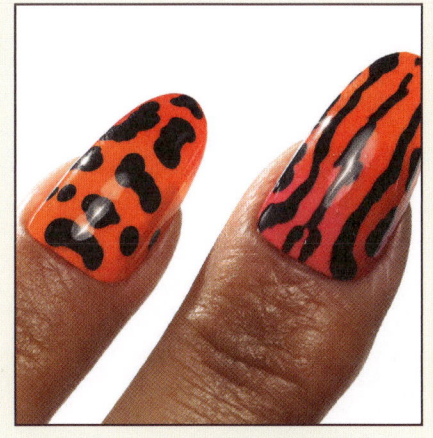

Hands-on Tutorials

145

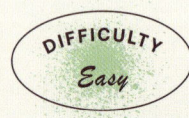

Stamping plates

TIME
20 MIN

So, you're not so great at the tedious stuff? Not to worry, there's a super simple way to achieve just about any amount of detail or design with ease. These were, in a lot of ways, the origin story to much of my nail collection and over 15 years later I still own my original stamping plate. The technique hasn't changed and neither has the pay-off!

WHAT YOU'LL NEED

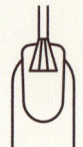 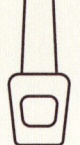 × 2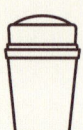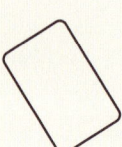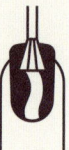

METHOD

① Apply your base coat.

② Apply your base colour.

③ Apply a swipe of your preferred design colour on one side of your chosen design. Stamping polishes do have the best consistency to ensure a neat design, however if you're using regular polish, the thicker and more pigmented, the better.

④ At an angle and with even pressure swipe the excess polish with a scraper.

⑤ Firmly and in one motion, press the stamp onto the stamping plate.

⑥ Check the stamp to ensure the polish has been evenly distributed across the design. If your design doesn't look even on the stamp, wipe off the stamp and plate with nail polish remover or acetone, wait for it to evaporate and repeat step 3, 4 and 5 again.

⑦ With an even pressure, press the stamp onto the nail and ensure the stamp has pressed evenly into the sides of the nail.

⑧ Once dry apply your top coat.

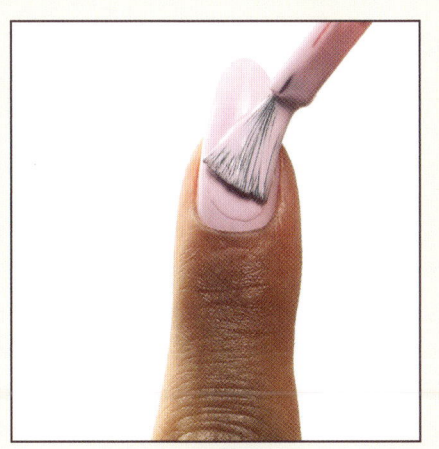
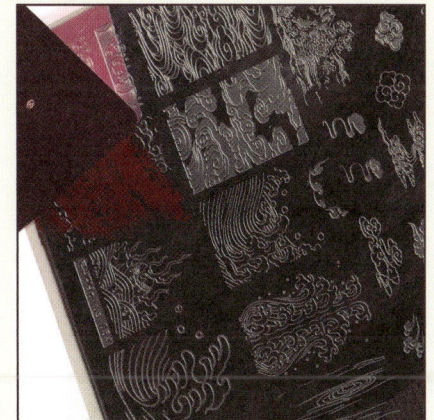
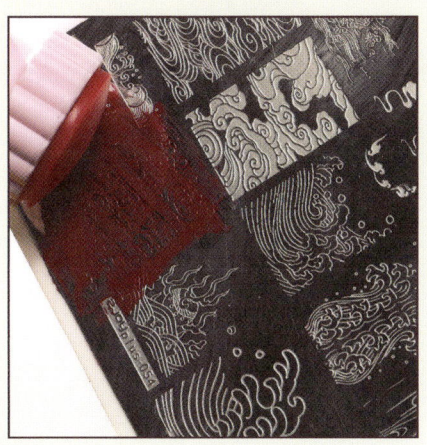
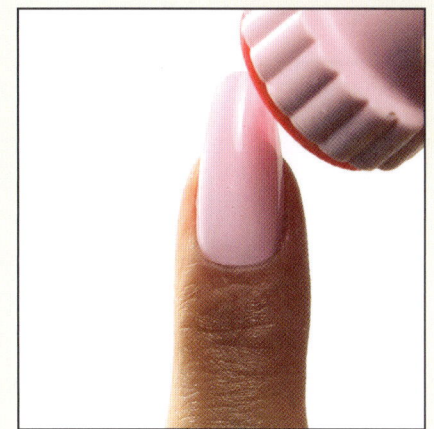
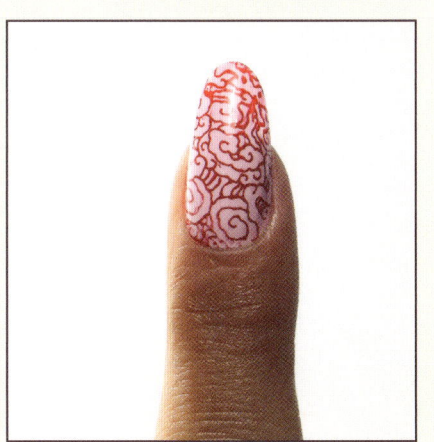
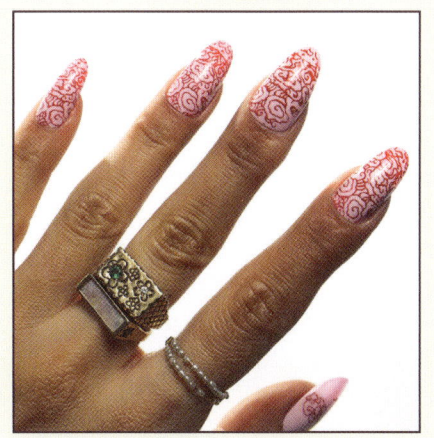

Hands-on Tutorials

147

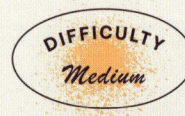

Alien shapes

TIME
20 MIN

Organic shapes and forms have always appealed to my eye and that's no different on nails. They're playful, easy to create, unique on each nail and any misstep is a little fun addition. No mistakes here!

WHAT YOU'LL NEED

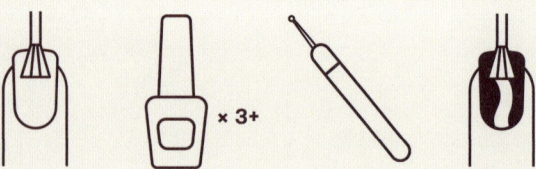

STEPS

① Apply your base coat.

② Apply your base colour. I love a glitter or speckled polish to give added dimension to the organic shapes.

③ Place random dots over the nail with a dotting tool and then join them with thinner lines.

④ Once dry, apply another colour in the widest points of the shape.

⑤ Repeat step 4 with as many colours as you please to create dimension. Contrast really adds to the look!

⑥ Once dry apply your top coat.

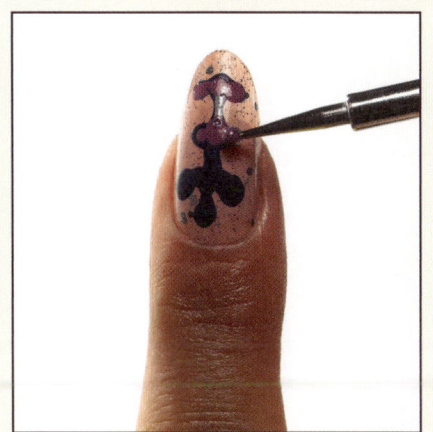
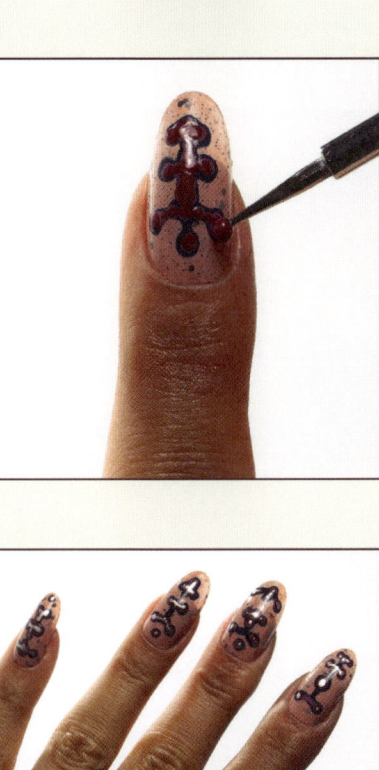
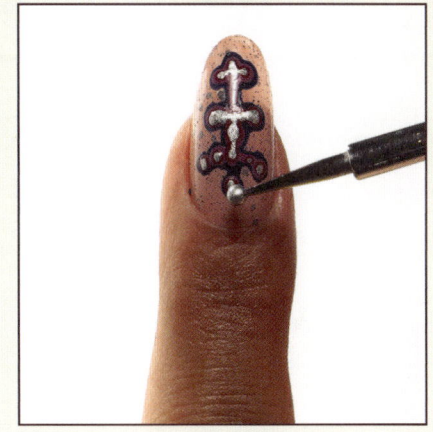
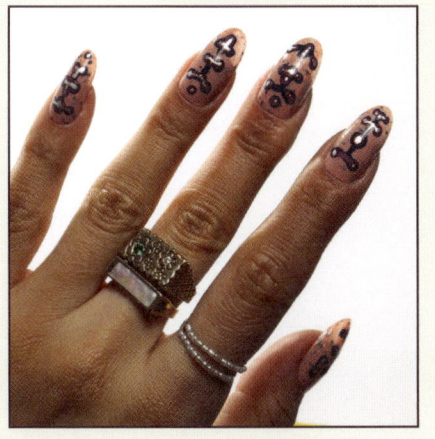
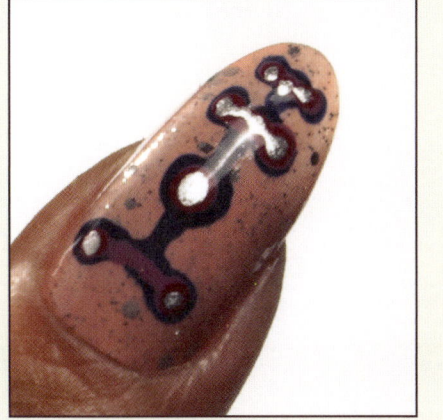

Hands-on Tutorials

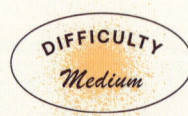

Watermarbling

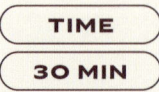

All trends come back around in a cycle and if there's any childhood nail look that I think should make a return it's water marbling. It's playful, dynamic and can be super detailed too!

WHAT YOU'LL NEED

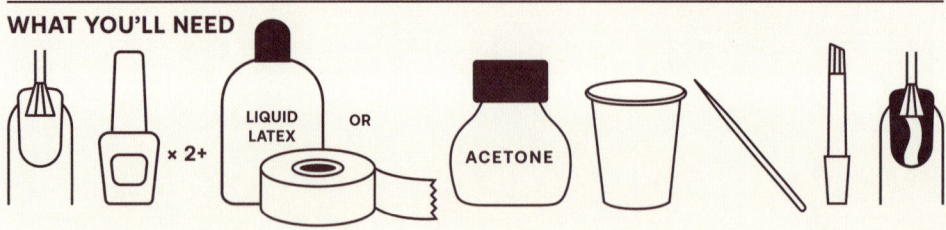

METHOD

① Apply your base coat.

② Apply liquid latex or tape around the tip of your finger.

③ Set up a disposable cup of room temperature water. Bottled or filtered water is best as it helps the polish spread.

④ Drip a drop of polish into the water.

⑤ Repeat step 4 in multiple colours until you've achieved your desired look. Move quickly as you still want to be able to manipulate the shapes in the cup before the polish hardens.

⑥ Using a toothpick, drag across the polish in the cup to create your desired pattern.

⑦ Lower your finger into the water as flat as possible.

⑧ While leaving your finger in the water, swirl the tooth pick around in the remaining polish to collect all remnants.

⑨ Lift your finger out only once the water is clear to avoid ruining the design on your nail.

⑩ With an angled brush lightly dipped in nail polish remover, clean up the edge of the nail.

⑪ Once dry apply your top coat.

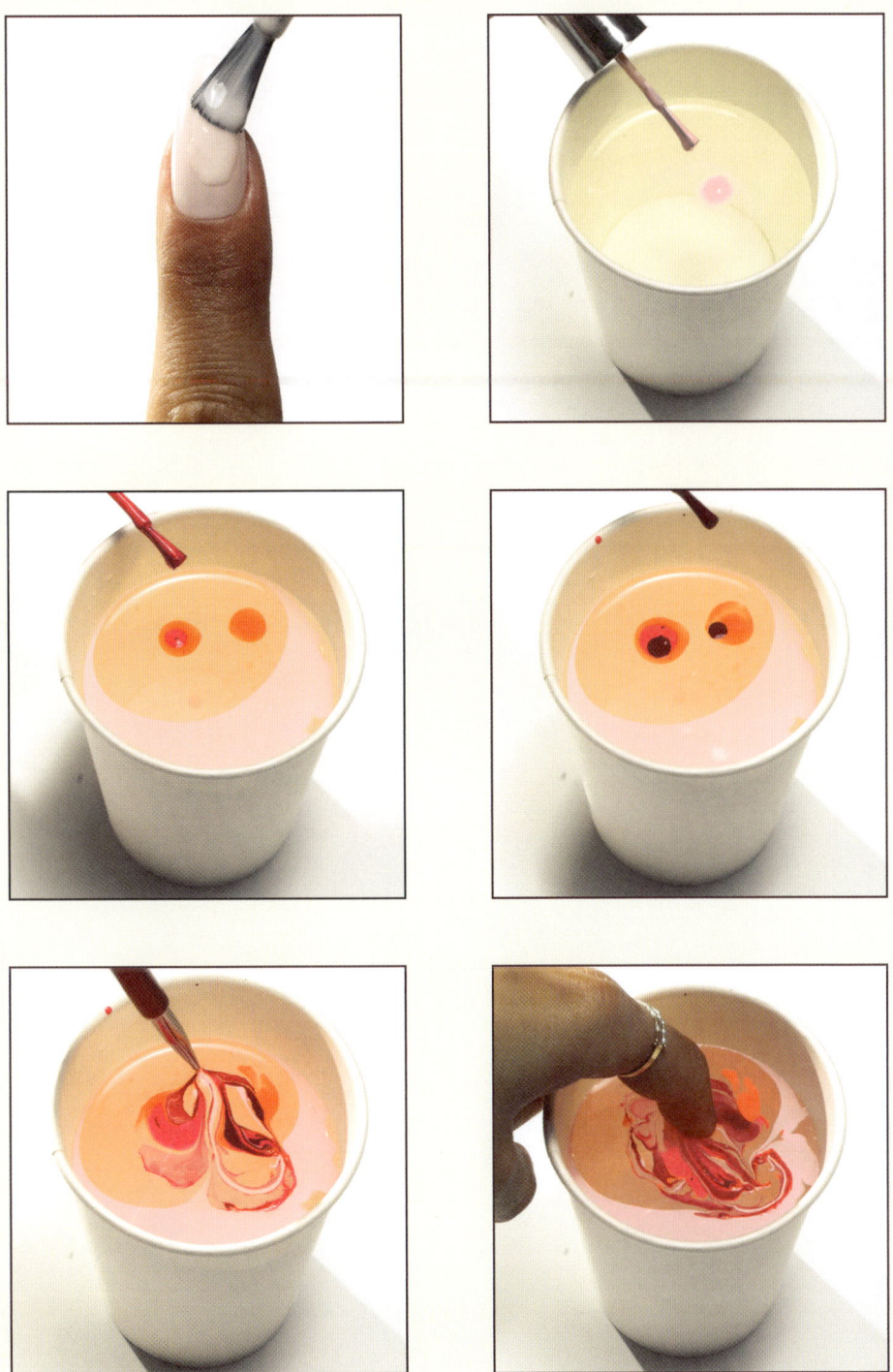

Hands-on Tutorials

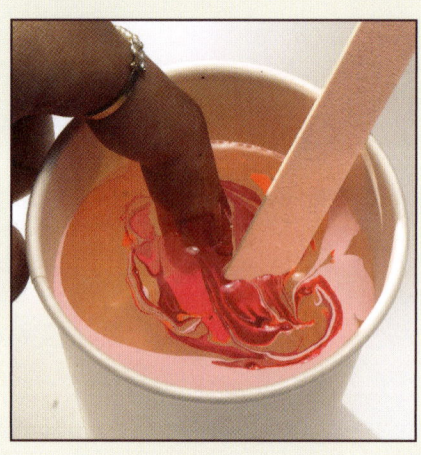
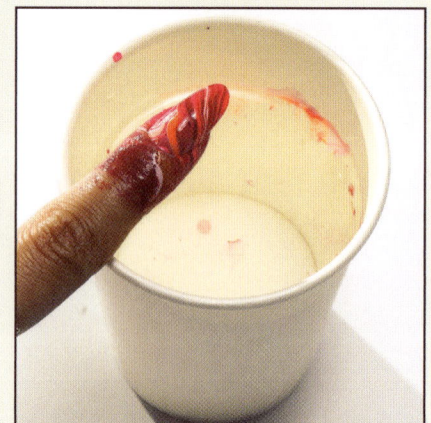
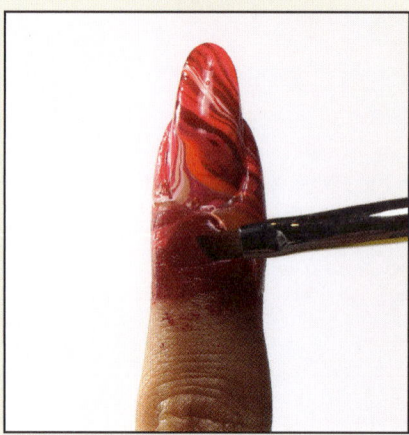
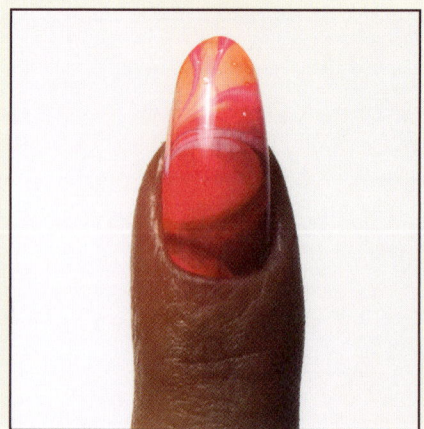

Mannequin Hands

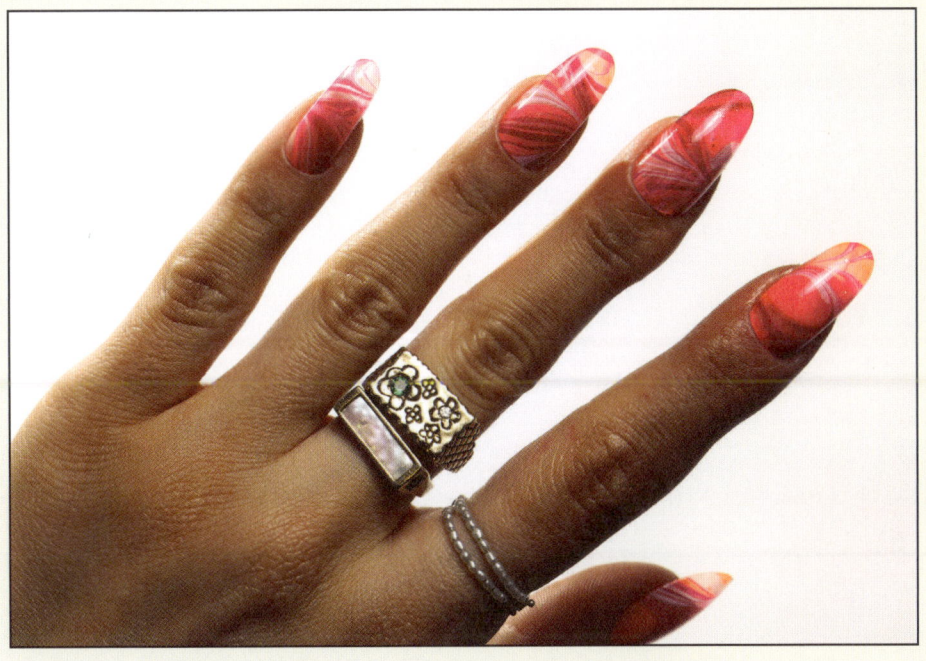

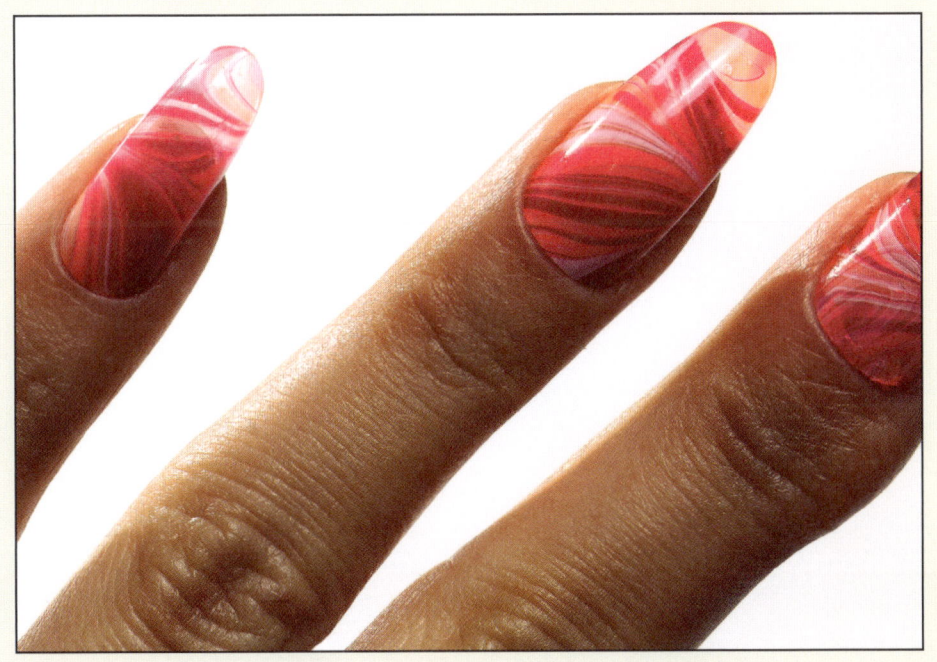

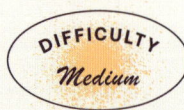

Texta scribbles

TIME
15 MIN

+

This is one of those techniques that you can really make the most of. It doesn't require you to work quickly like full polish designs do and you don't have to have much more than your marker to create a unique and fun design.

WHAT YOU'LL NEED

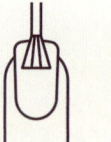 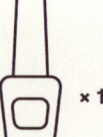 ×1 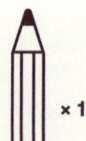 ×1+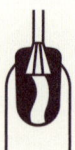

METHOD

① Apply your base coat.

② Apply your base colour. White or lighter colours are ideal as they ensure you get the greatest colour pay-off from your texta designs.

③ Once the base coat has completely dried, draw on your desired designs. This time I went with a bow, starting from one side of the nail into the centre to ensure balanced placement.

④ Once dry, apply any shading or details you like, for this set I applied a little dot in the centre of the bows.

⑤ Once dry apply your top coat.

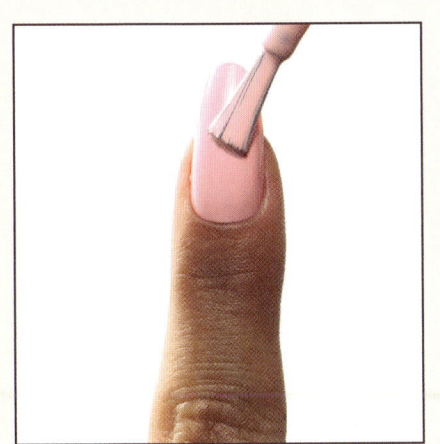
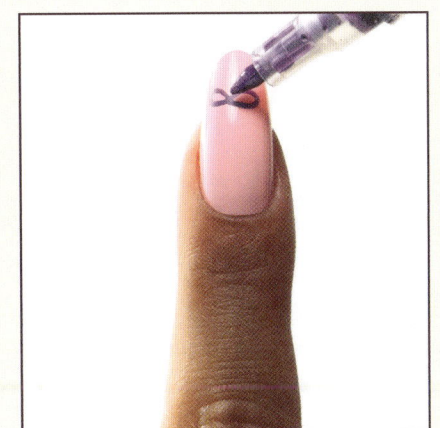
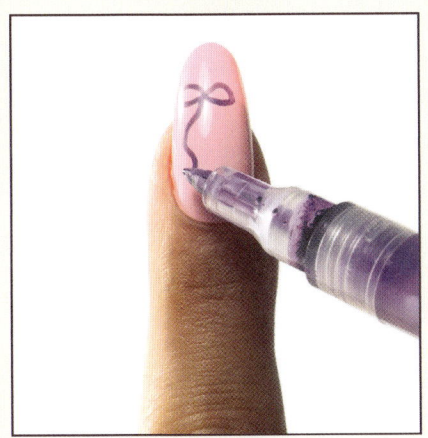
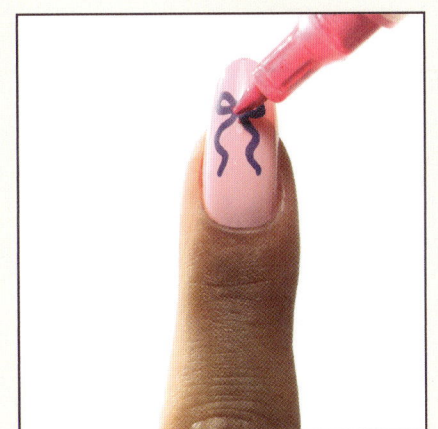
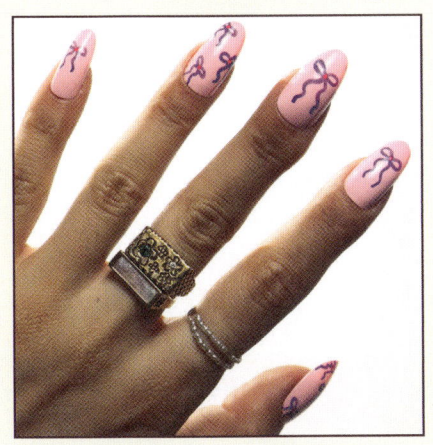
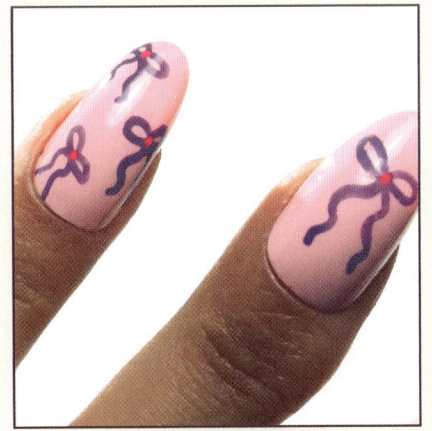

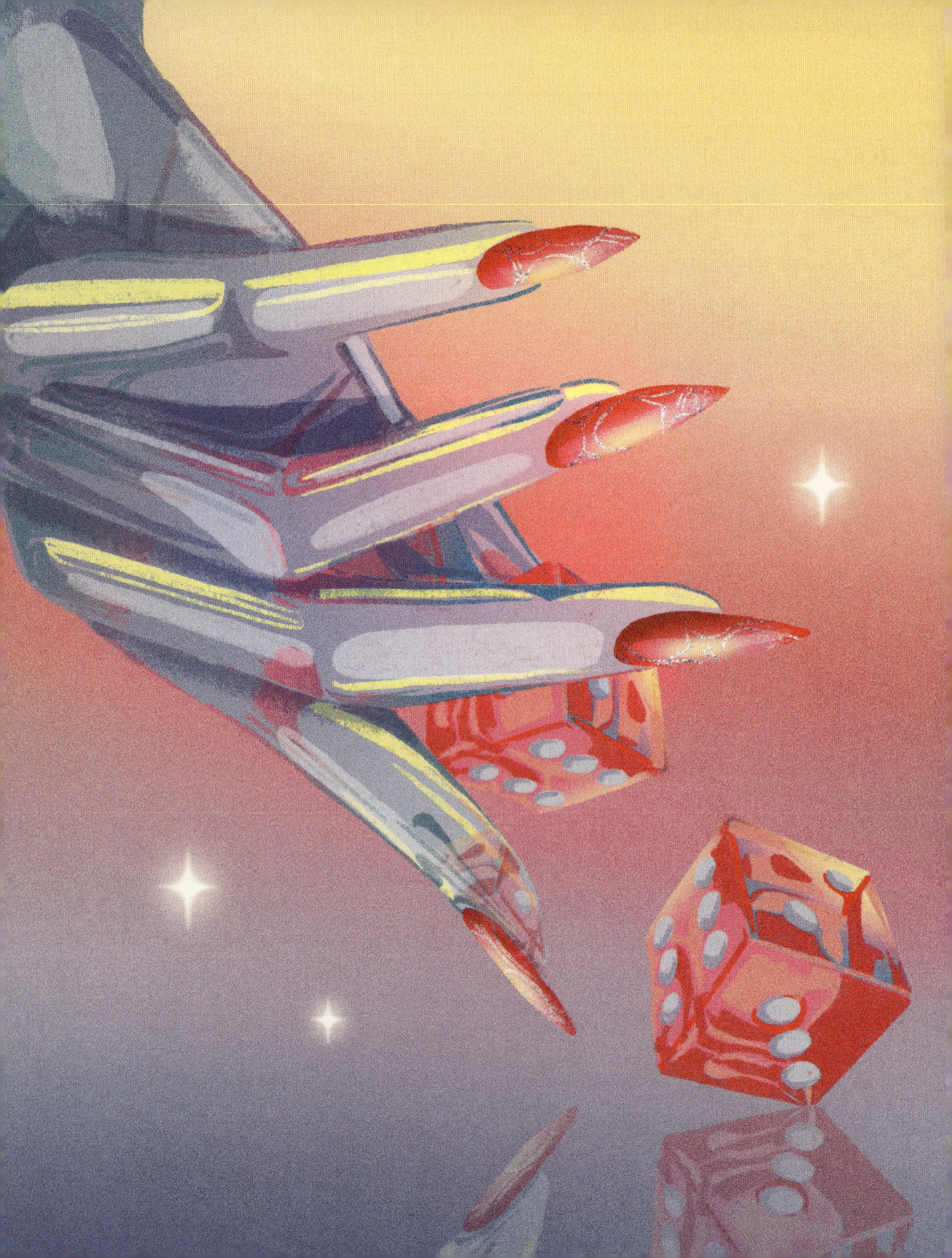

CHAPTER

STICK IT

FIVE

PRESS-ON NAILS

Press-ons are the old underdog of the nail world. Previously limited to maybe three colours and a glitter made with super cheap, overly flexible tips that would inevitably crack in half in the middle of a dancefloor or emerge in the corner of your bathroom when you were none the wiser that you had one missing, the press-on has evolved, matured even.

It'd be hard to pinpoint exactly when this happened but we're glad it did. You could probably thank the global shut down of salons through covid-19 for their rise in popularity, but nurses, drag queens, actors and Halloween lovers have long loved the press-on.

Now, press-ons come in a range of quality, and plenty of luxurious, hand-crafted press-ons are made by nail techs all over the world. They can even be worn again if they're removed gently making them a cost-effective option too! They're perfect for daylong shoots or weeklong wear depending on how they're applied.

HOW TO APPLY
Press-ons

① Wash and dry your hands.

② Push cuticles back with a cuticle pusher.

③ Buff the natural nail to remove any shine.

④ Wipe the nail bed with the alcohol wipe to clean.

⑤ Gently apply nail glue to the natural nail and to the press-on at the base of the nail at an angle, touch the press-on to the base of the nail then lower the press-on to the tip to ensure even application of the glue.

⑥ Hold the nail in place for 15 seconds.

⑦ Avoid washing your hands, applying creams or using chemicals for the next hour.

HOW TO REMOVE
Press-ons

① Apply cuticle oil generously to your cuticles.

② Soak your hands in warm soapy water until the glue dissolves.

③ Slide the press-on nails off without force.

④ If they absolutely won't budge and you're happy to sacrifice your press-ons they can be soaked off with acetone.

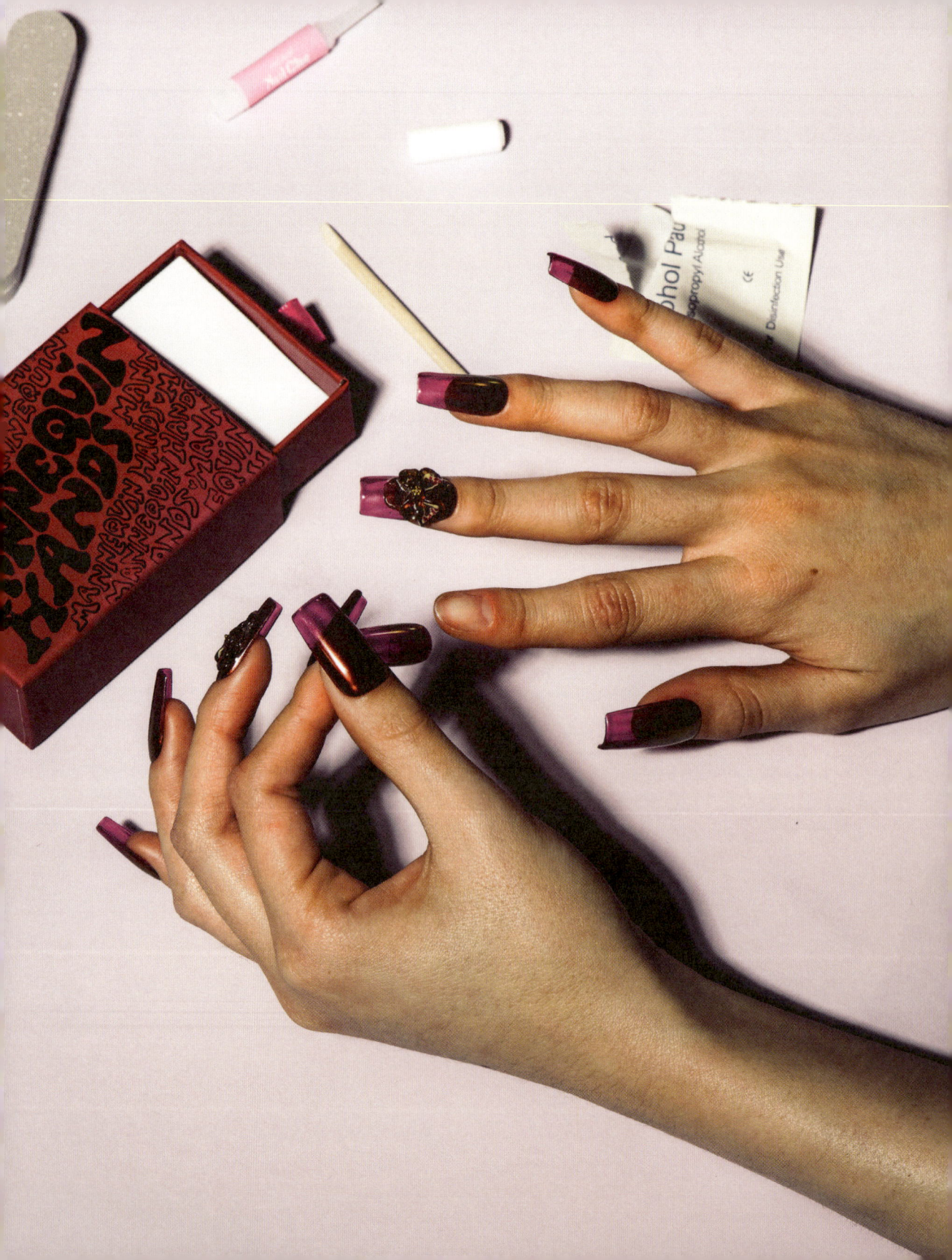

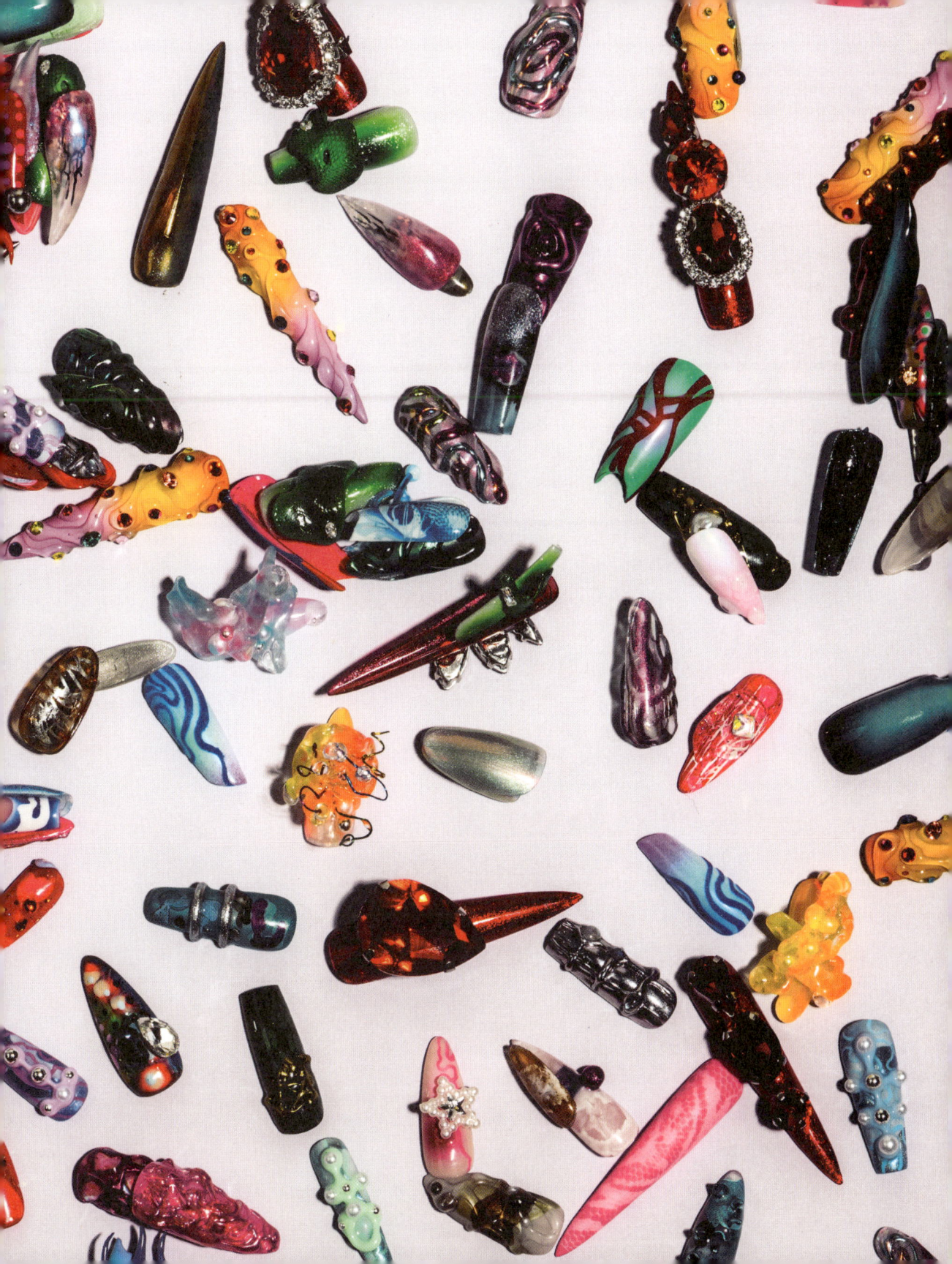

DECALS

All I've ever dreamed of is making as many people as possible love nail art in all the ways I do. If I could hold hands with everyone reading this and make nail art magic happen I would. But thankfully there's a perfect solution for the nail art loving world I long for! Attached is a selection of nail decals carefully curated for you. If you're a fan of nail art but not so good at executing fiddly designs yourself, it's time to meet nail decals. They're fun, they're easy and they're the perfect solution for adding detail to your nails in a matter of seconds.

I have curated a brand new set of nail decals, just for this book, so I can fulfil my goal of touching as many hands as possible. I made sure to include some of my most requested designs and some versatile basics like smiley faces, hearts and stars because there's no nail art set that wouldn't benefit from that playful touch. I hand-painted some of my signature linework that works perfectly worn solo, or even better layered over a bunch of different colours and looks. Art and fashion have always been huge inspirations in my work, so I've also put in a bunch of referential moments that add dimension to a set with ease.

Maybe your hand won't work the way you want it to, or you're contorting your fingers to get all the detail right, but it just isn't working, or you're rushing to a party and your fingers need to catch up with the outfit. Nail decals are an invitation to play! For some people, a plain nail with a decal or two is the perfect mood-lifting look, for others nail decals are the perfect way to replicate the sticker book collections of childhood.

Whatever drives you, grab some tweezers and apply these nail decals!

HOW TO USE
Nail Decals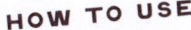

① Apply your coating of choice. Once dry, use tweezers to gently bend the plastic backing and pick the corner of your chosen decal off the sheet.

② Over a clean, dry surface gently place the nail decal in your desired spot.

③ Smooth the nail decal onto the nail from the centre outwards to ensure there are no creases or folds.

④ Apply your favourite top coat to seal in your design.

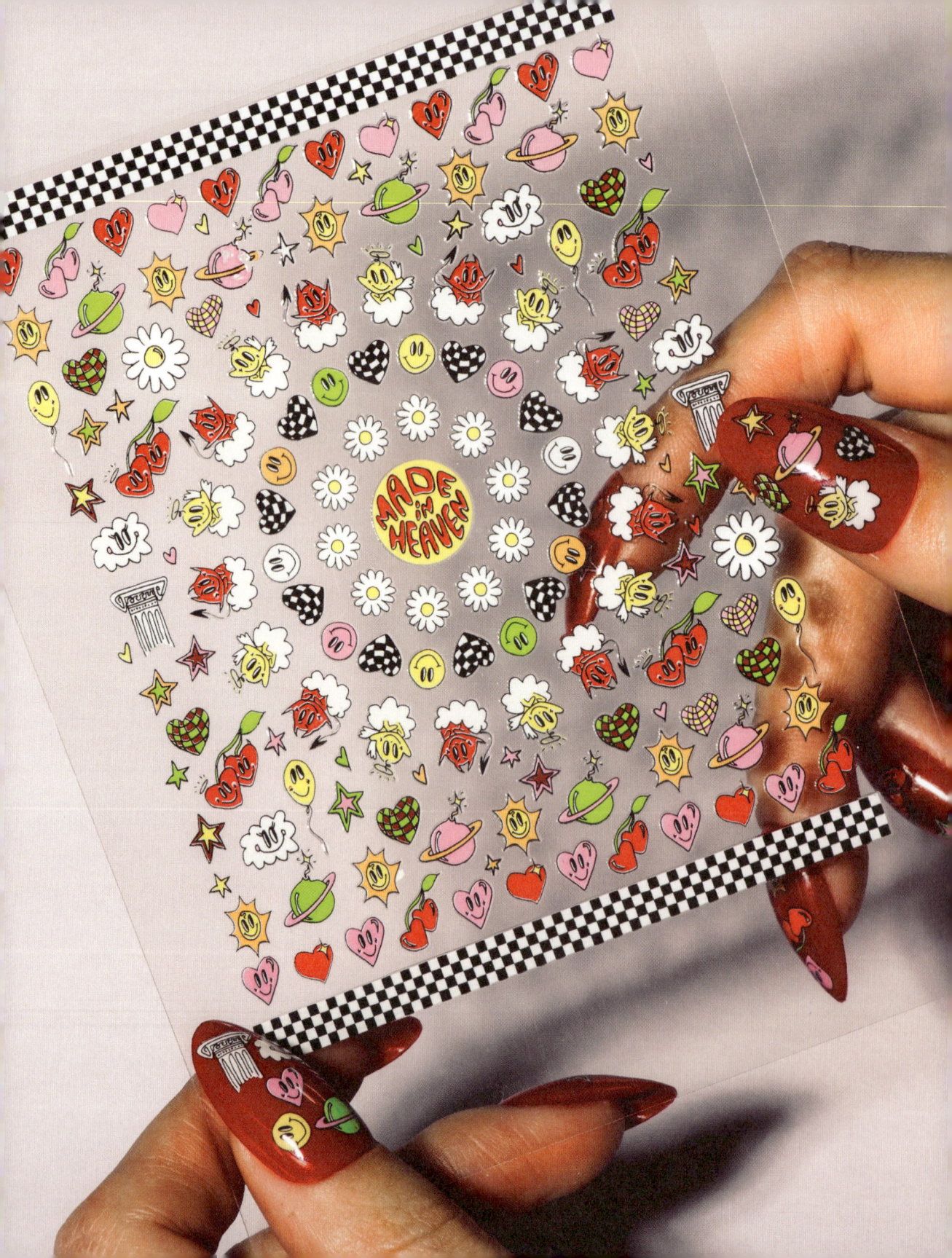

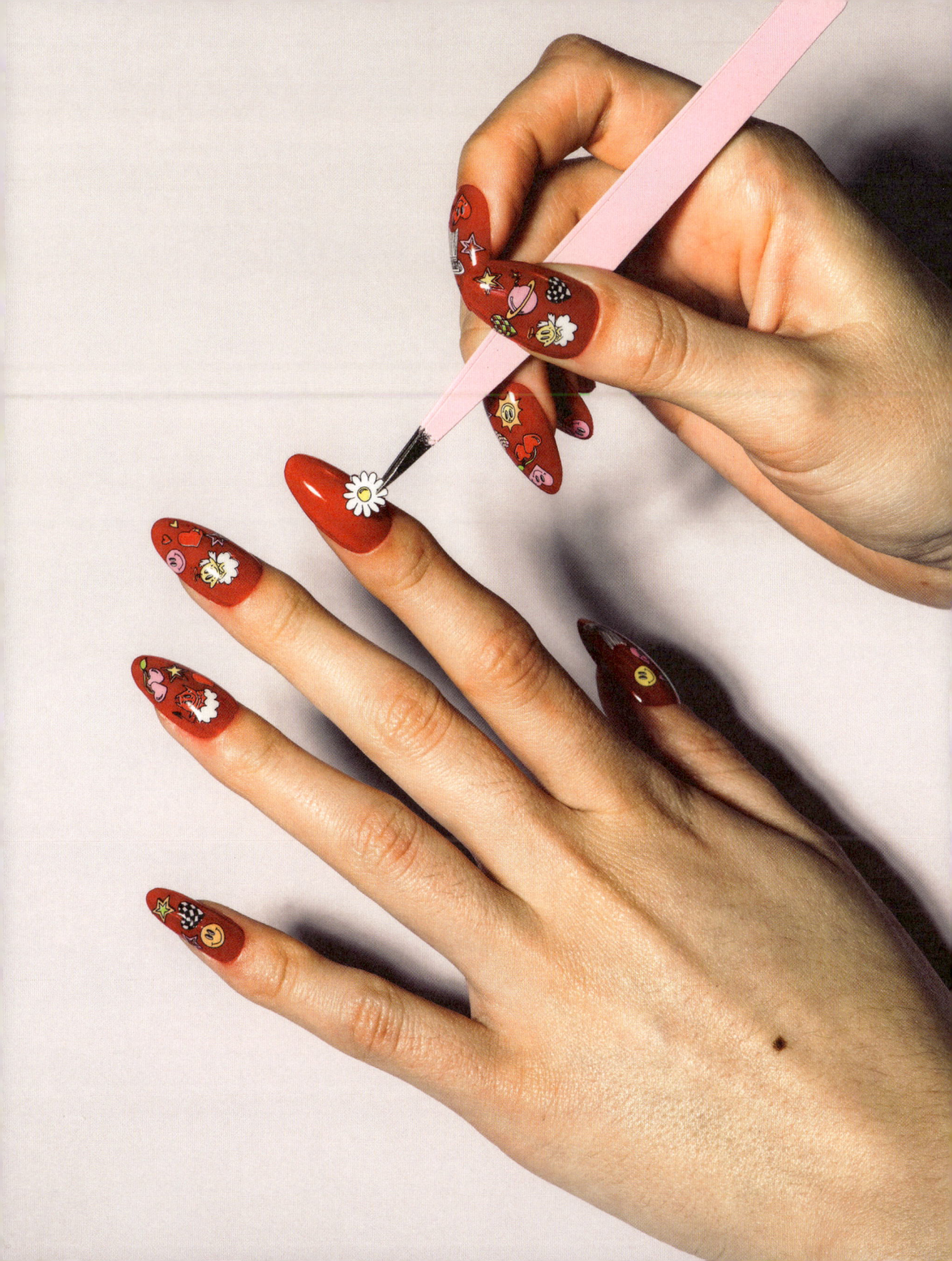

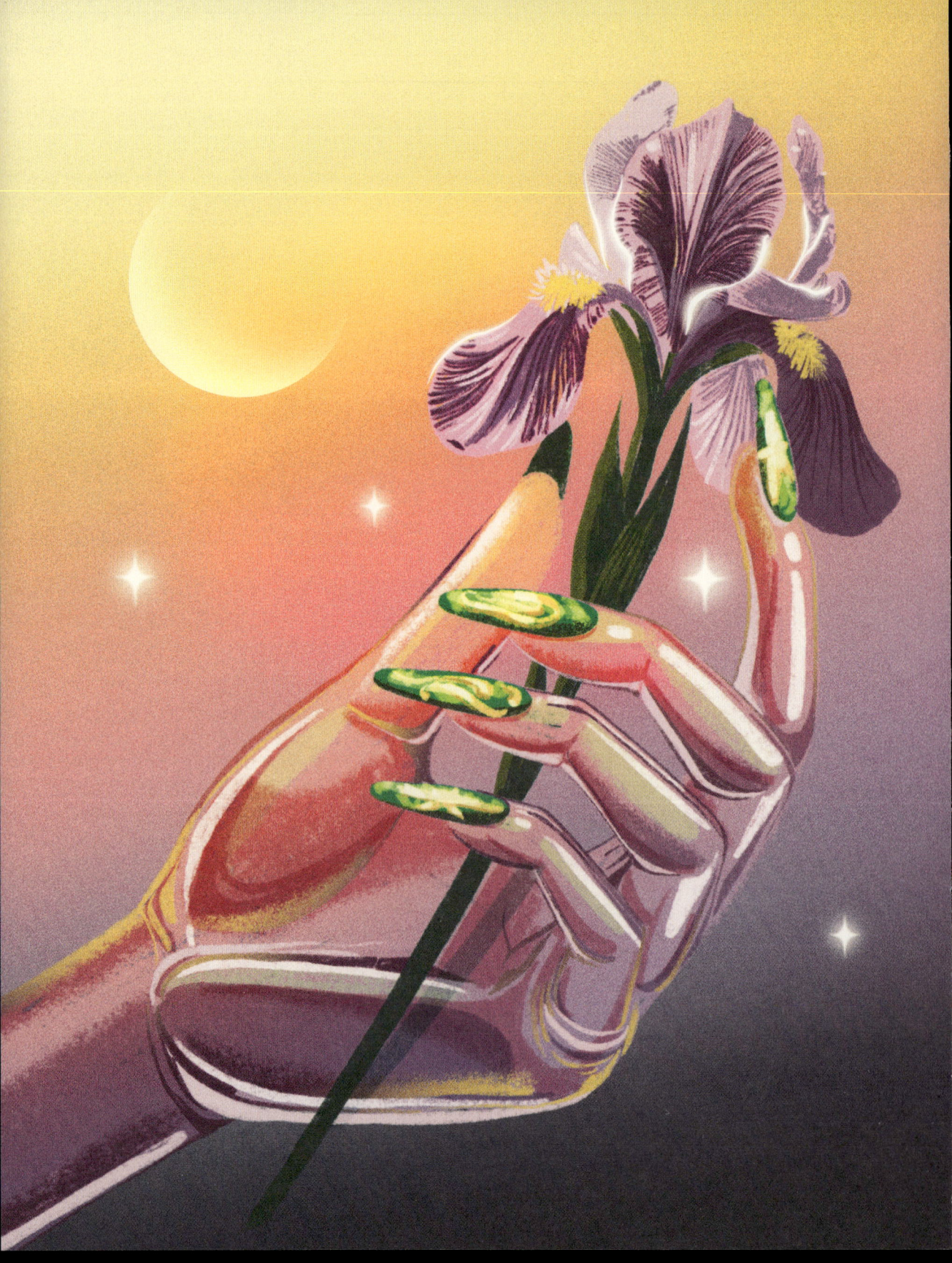

CHAPTER

CREATE IT

SIX

SKETCHBOOK

*A*ll I could ever hope is that this book inspires you to try out something new with your nails. Turn your bedroom into a nail salon or look at nail art as an art form in its own right. Art is nothing if it doesn't inspire creativity so for the rest of this book it's time to pour out all the things that your brain has conjured up with the nail art your eyes have lapped up.

Grab your pens, pencils, markers, watercolours, hell just about anything you can get to map out your most inspired nail art looks.

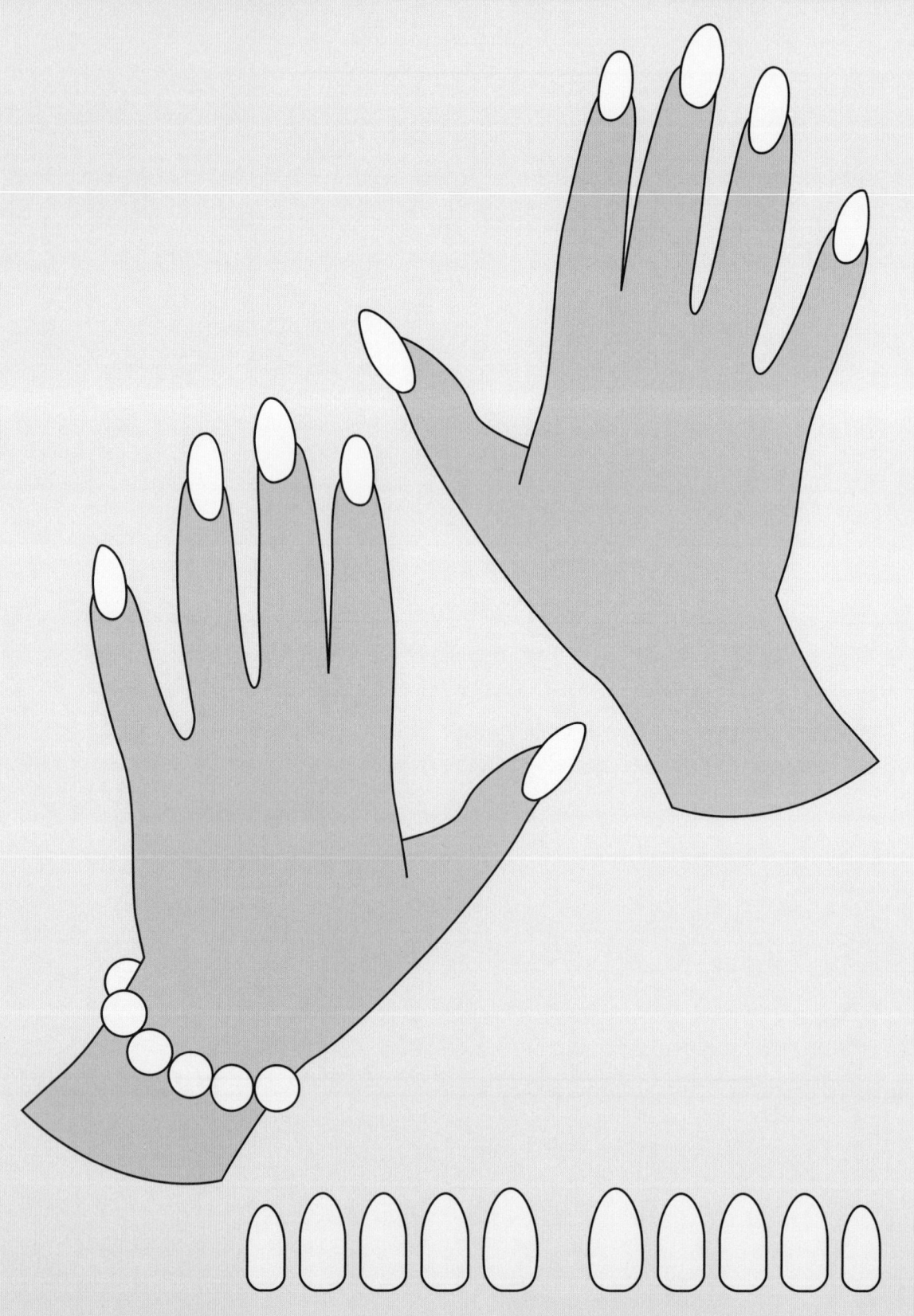

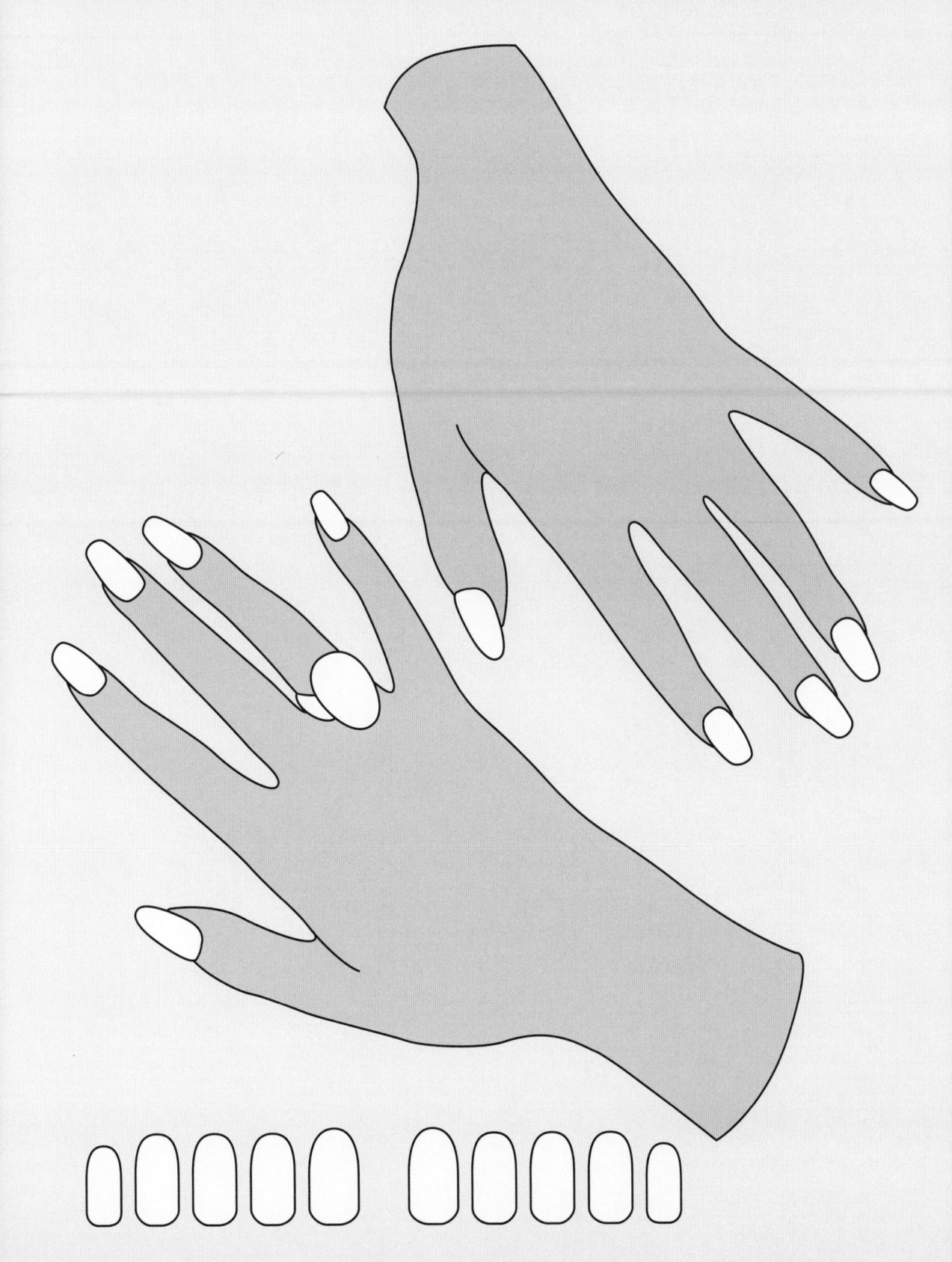

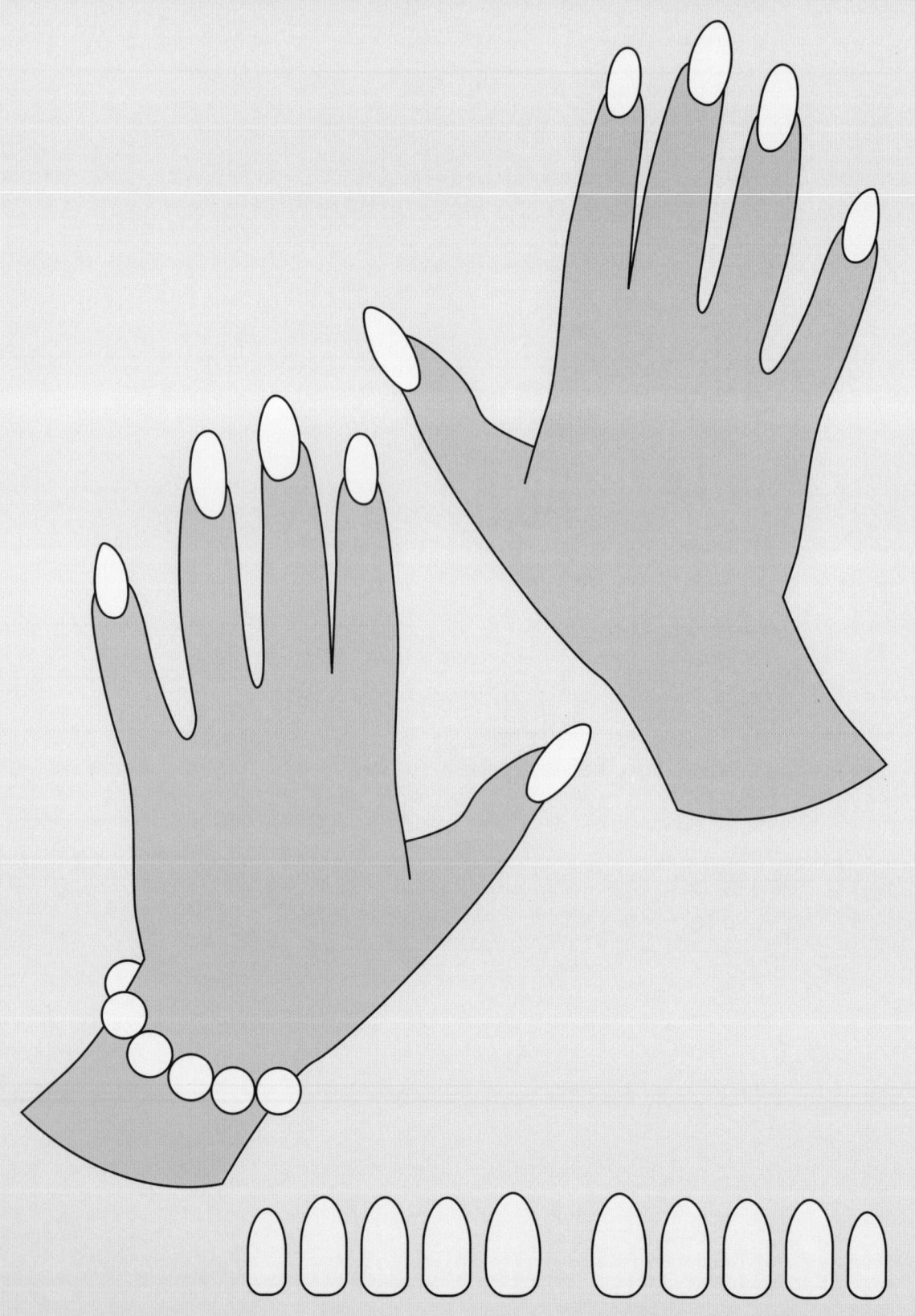

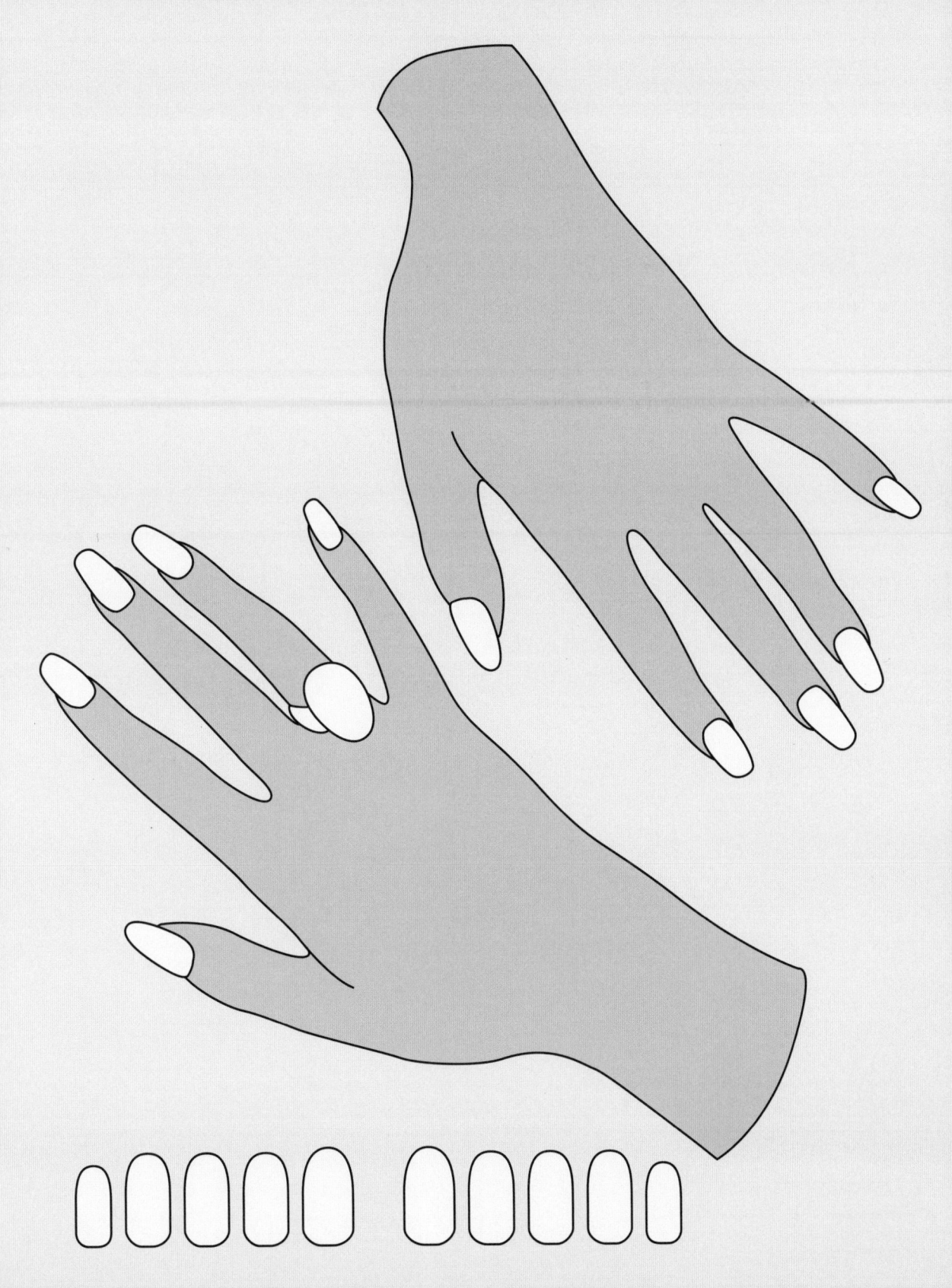

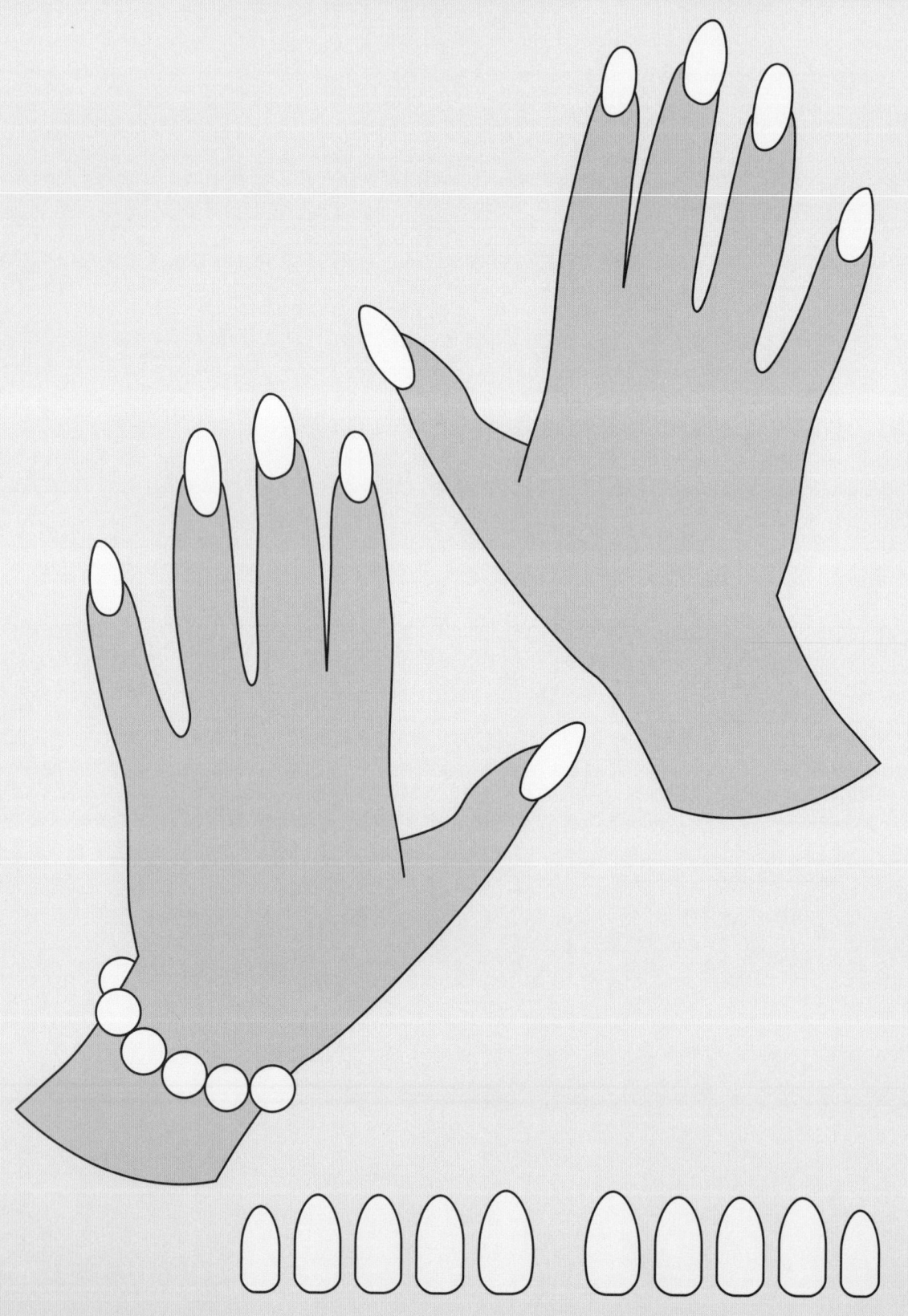

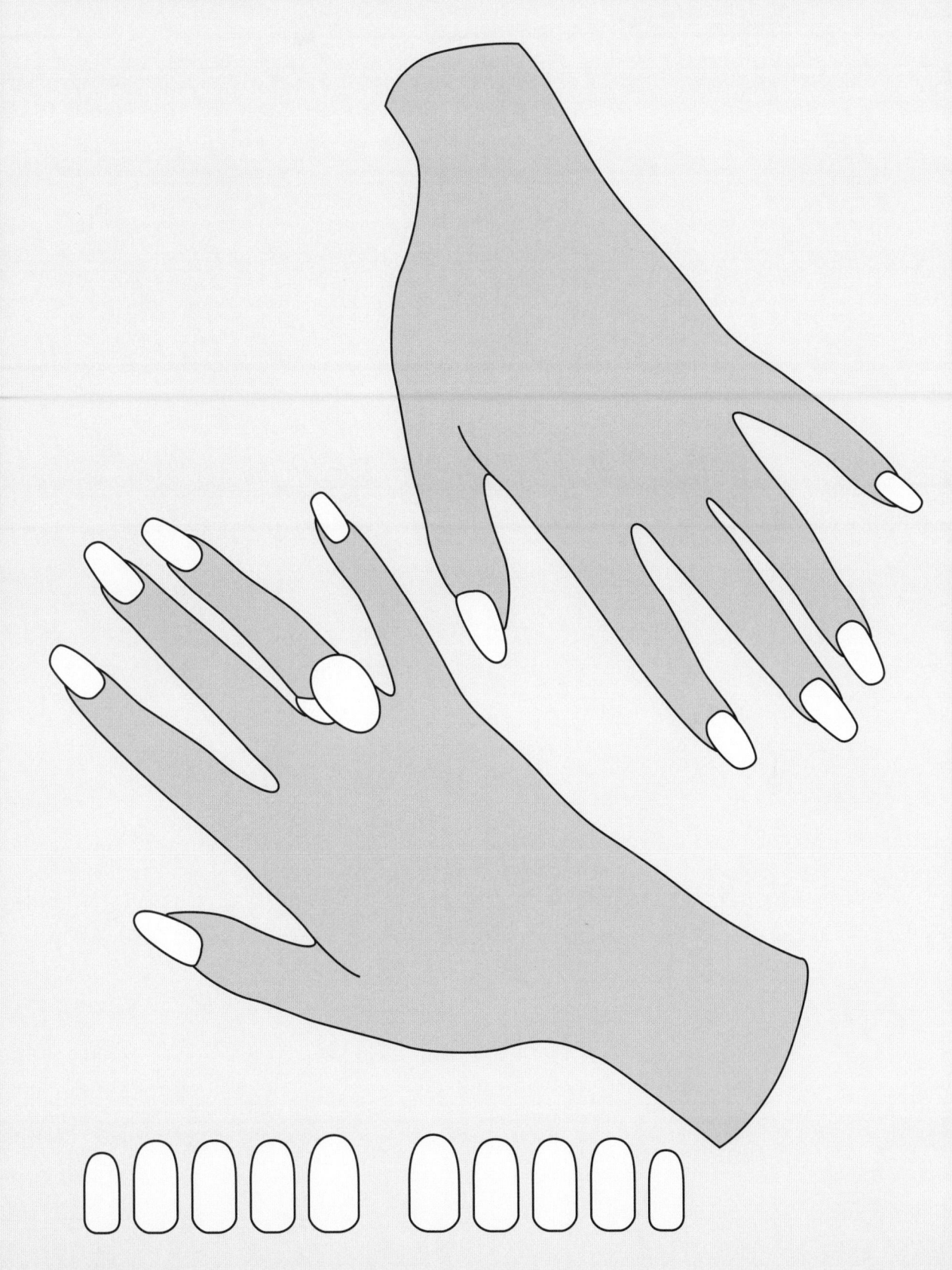

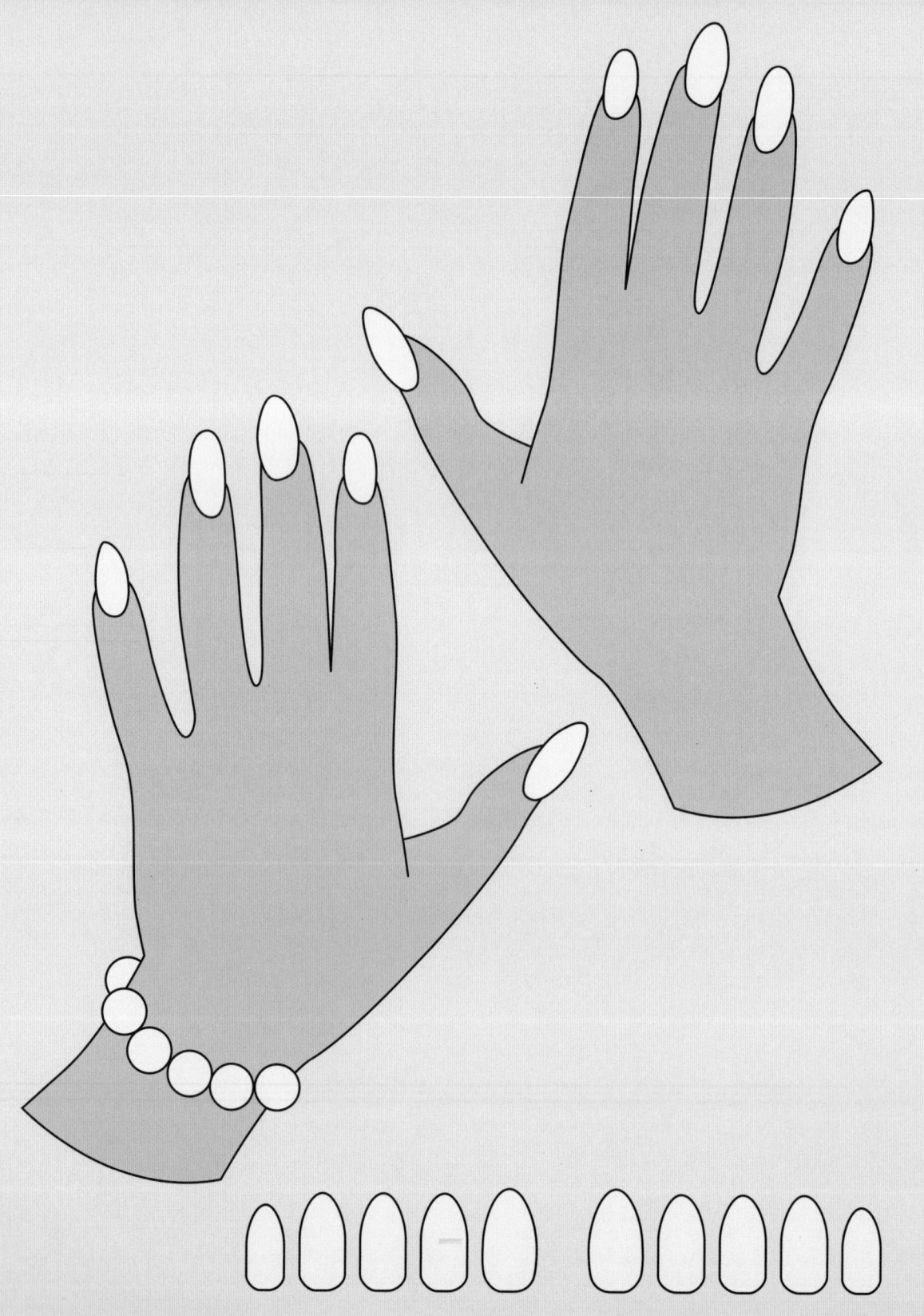

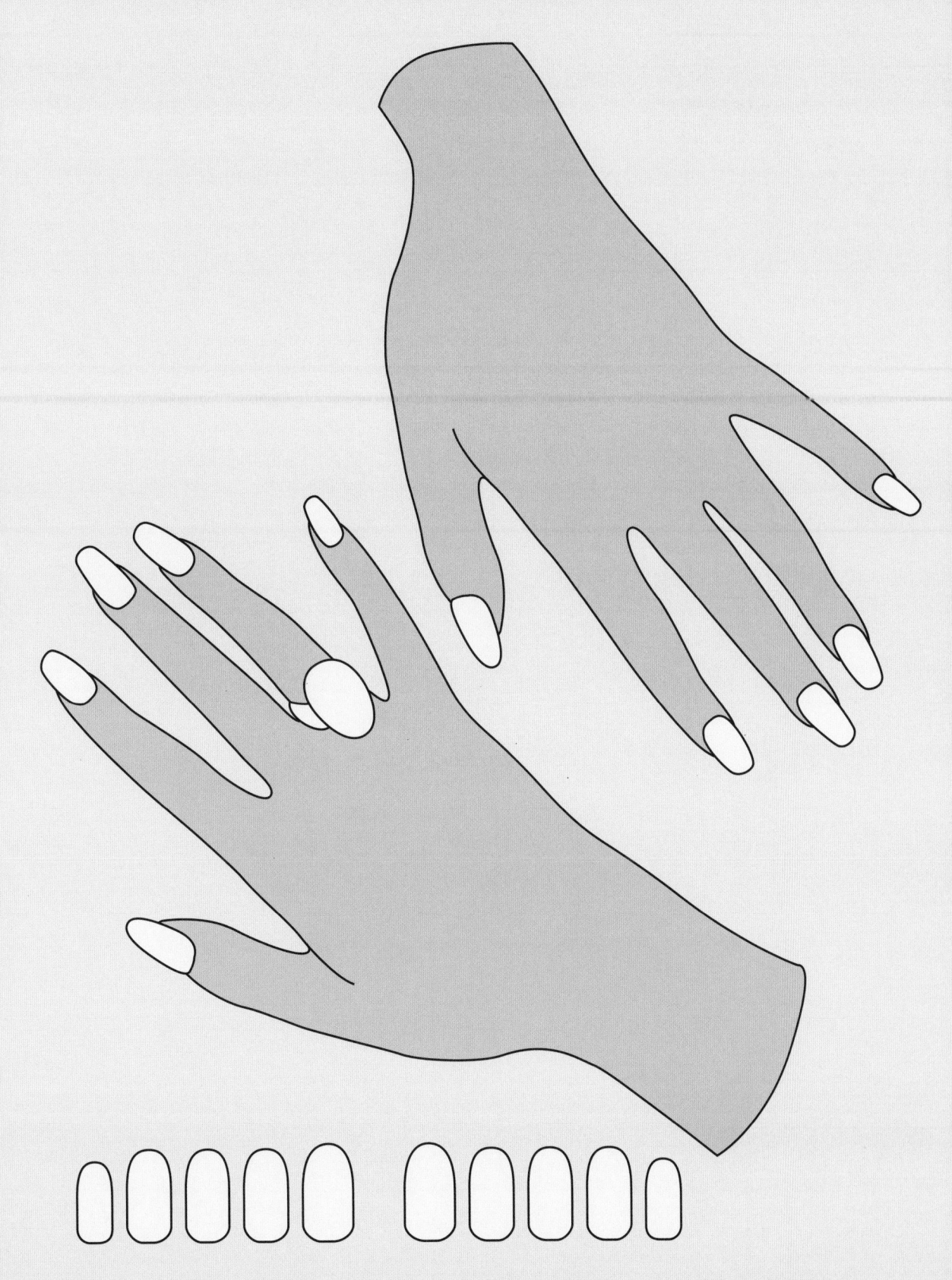

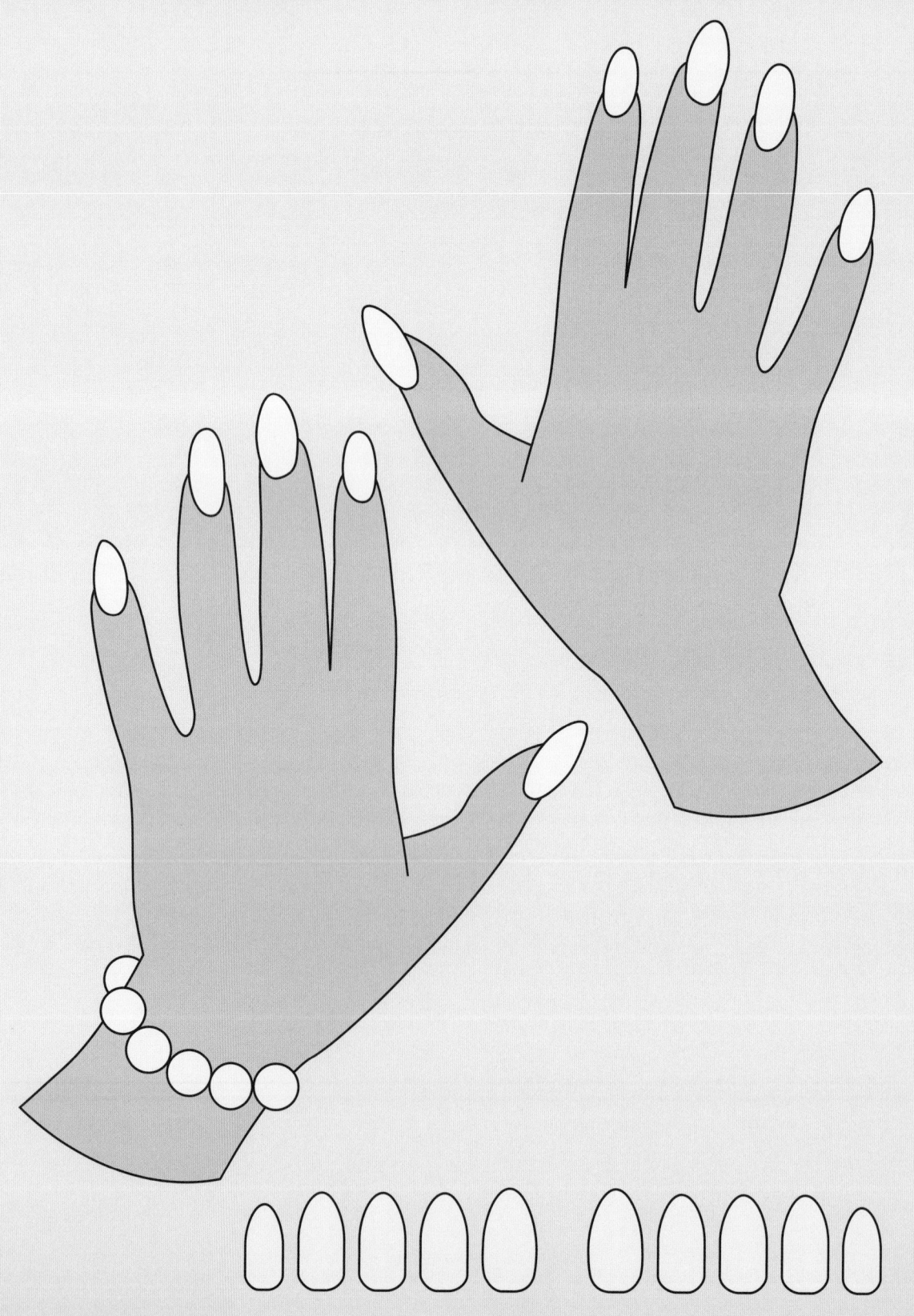

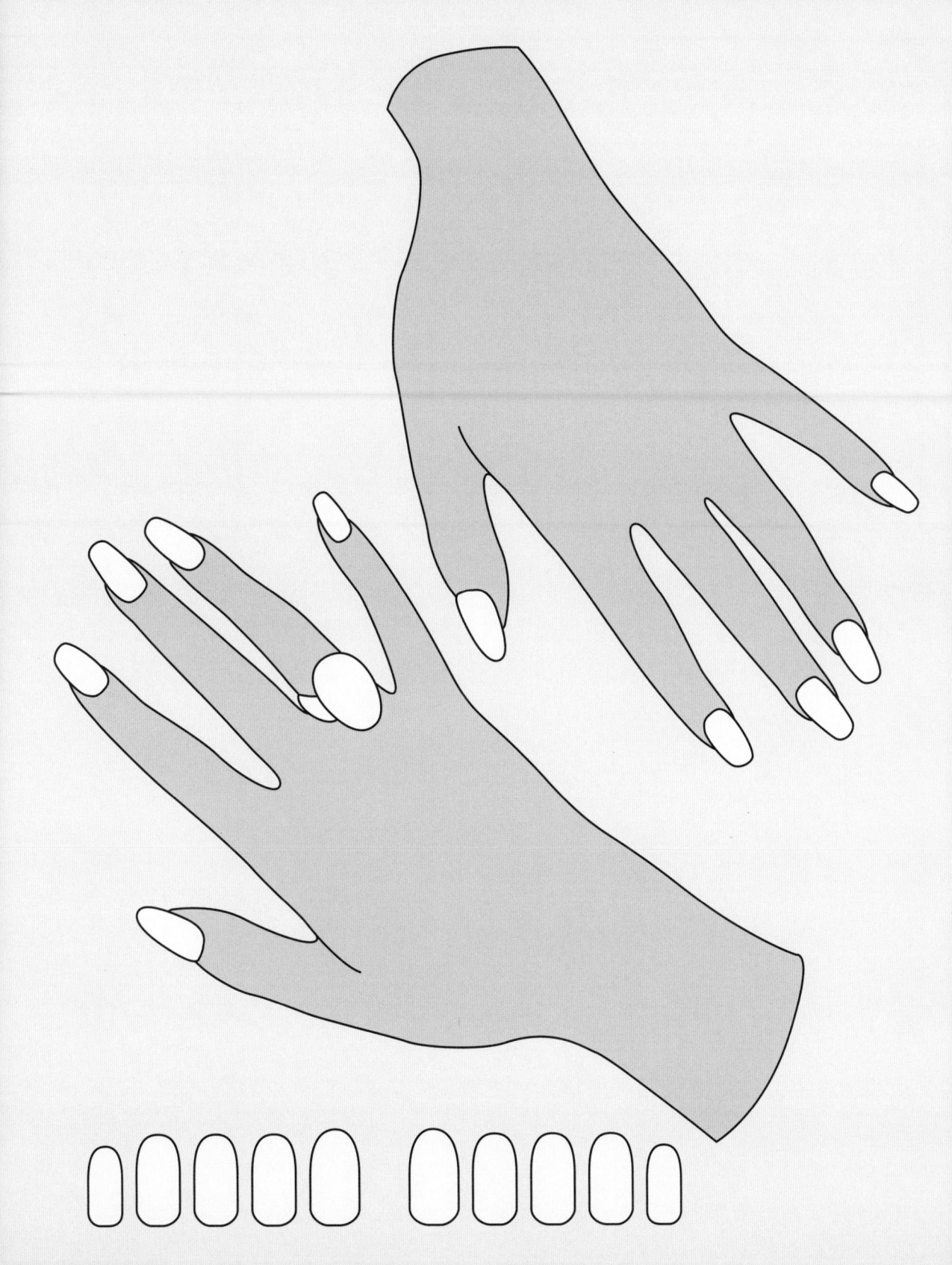

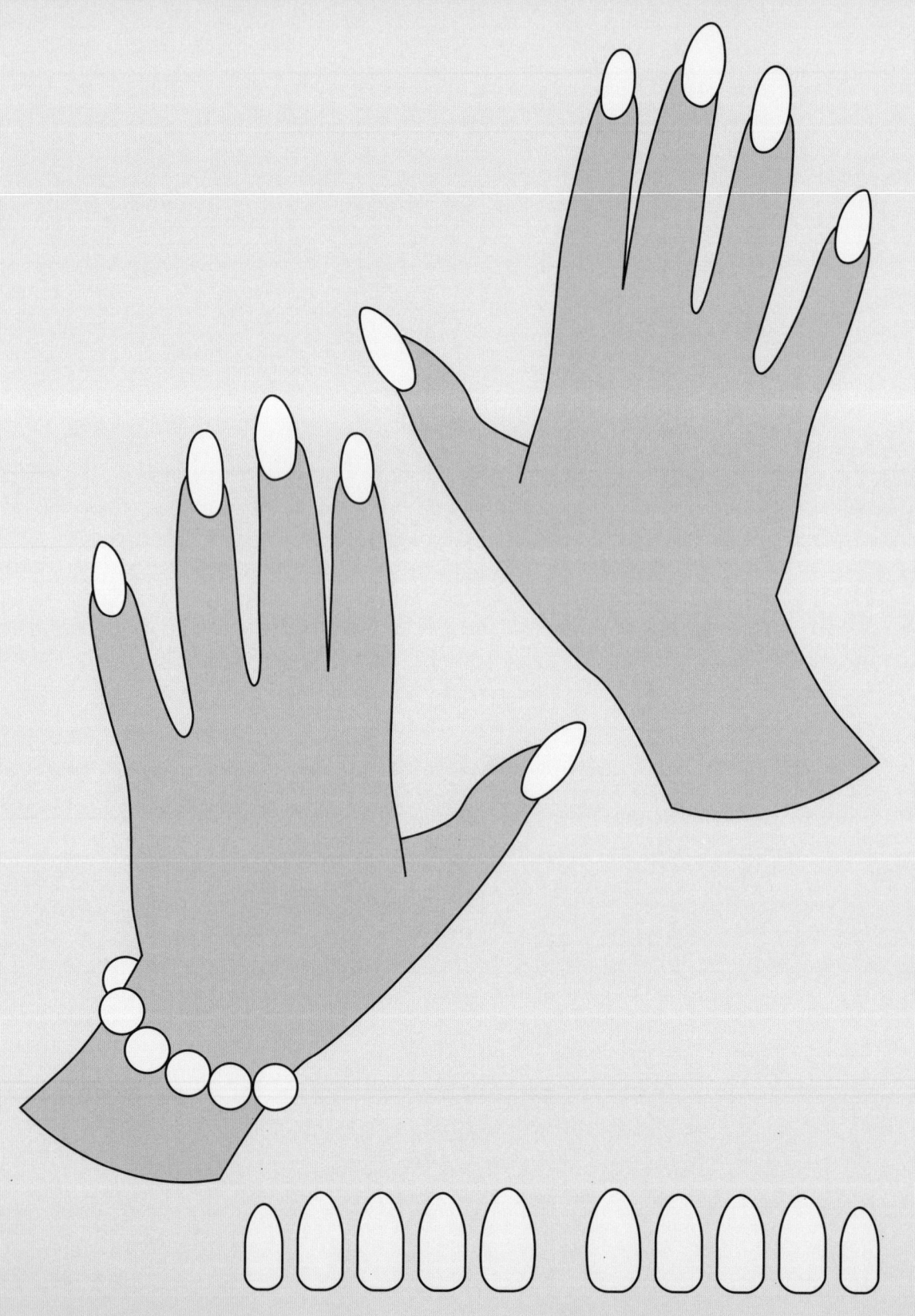

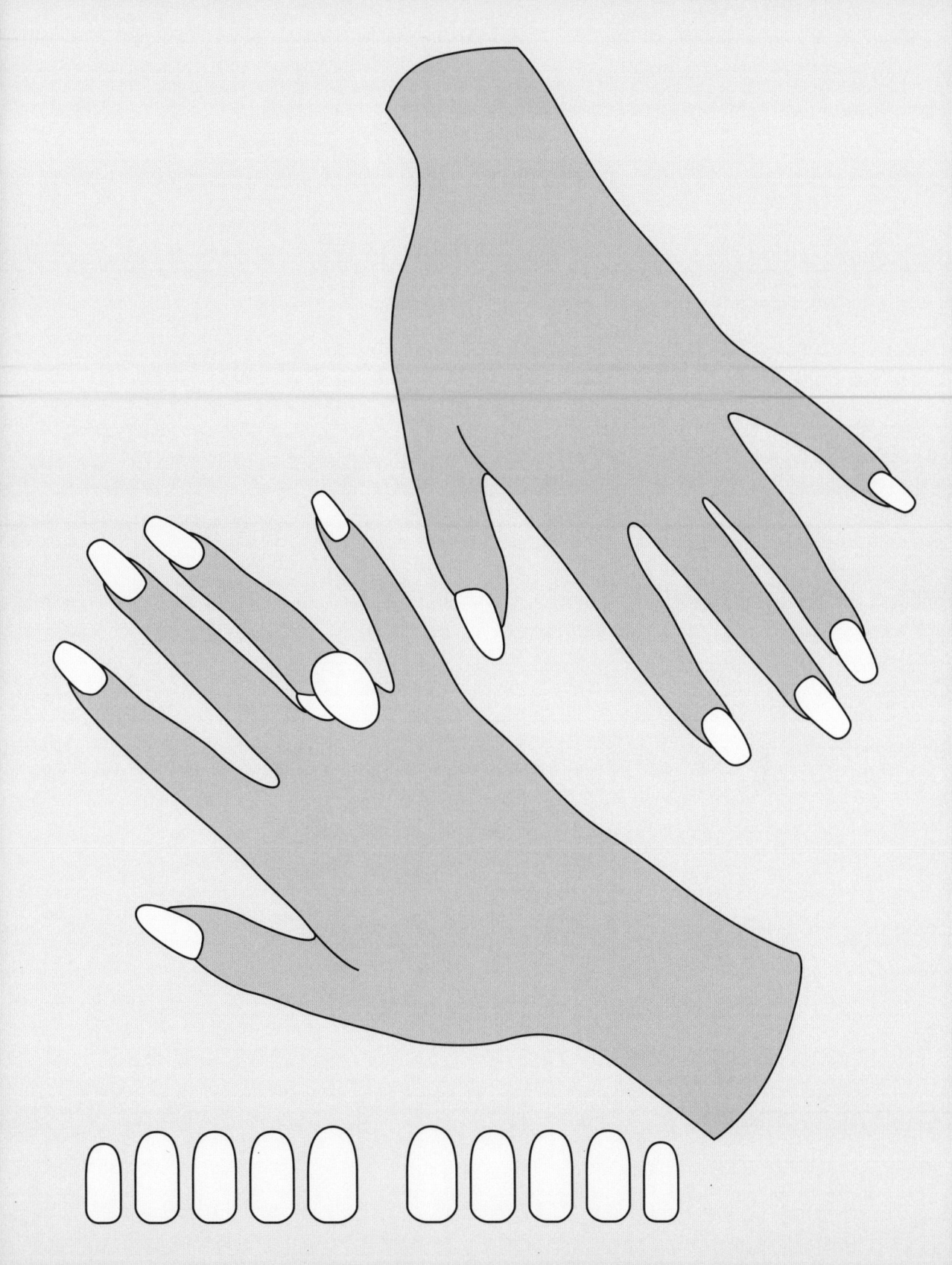

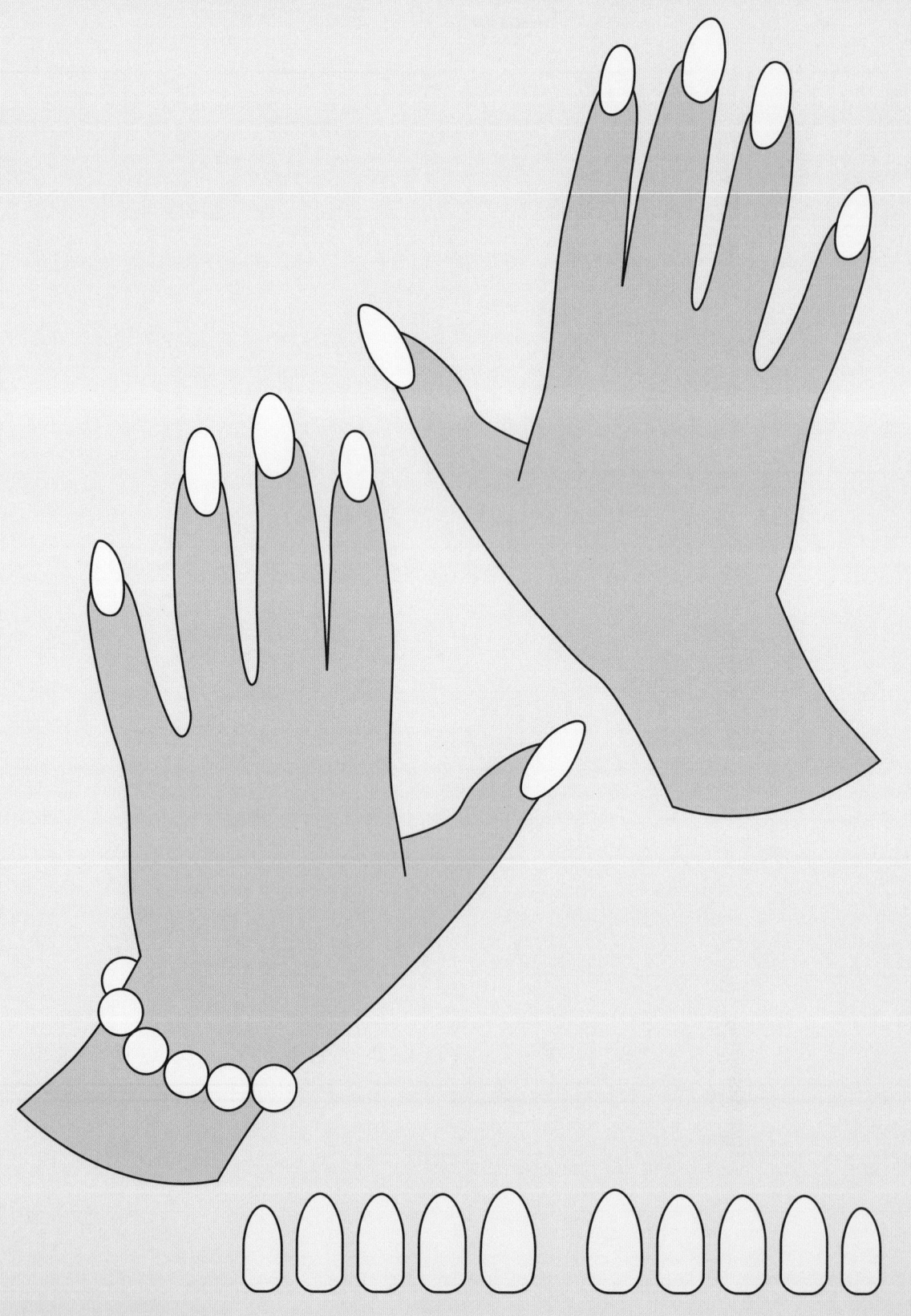

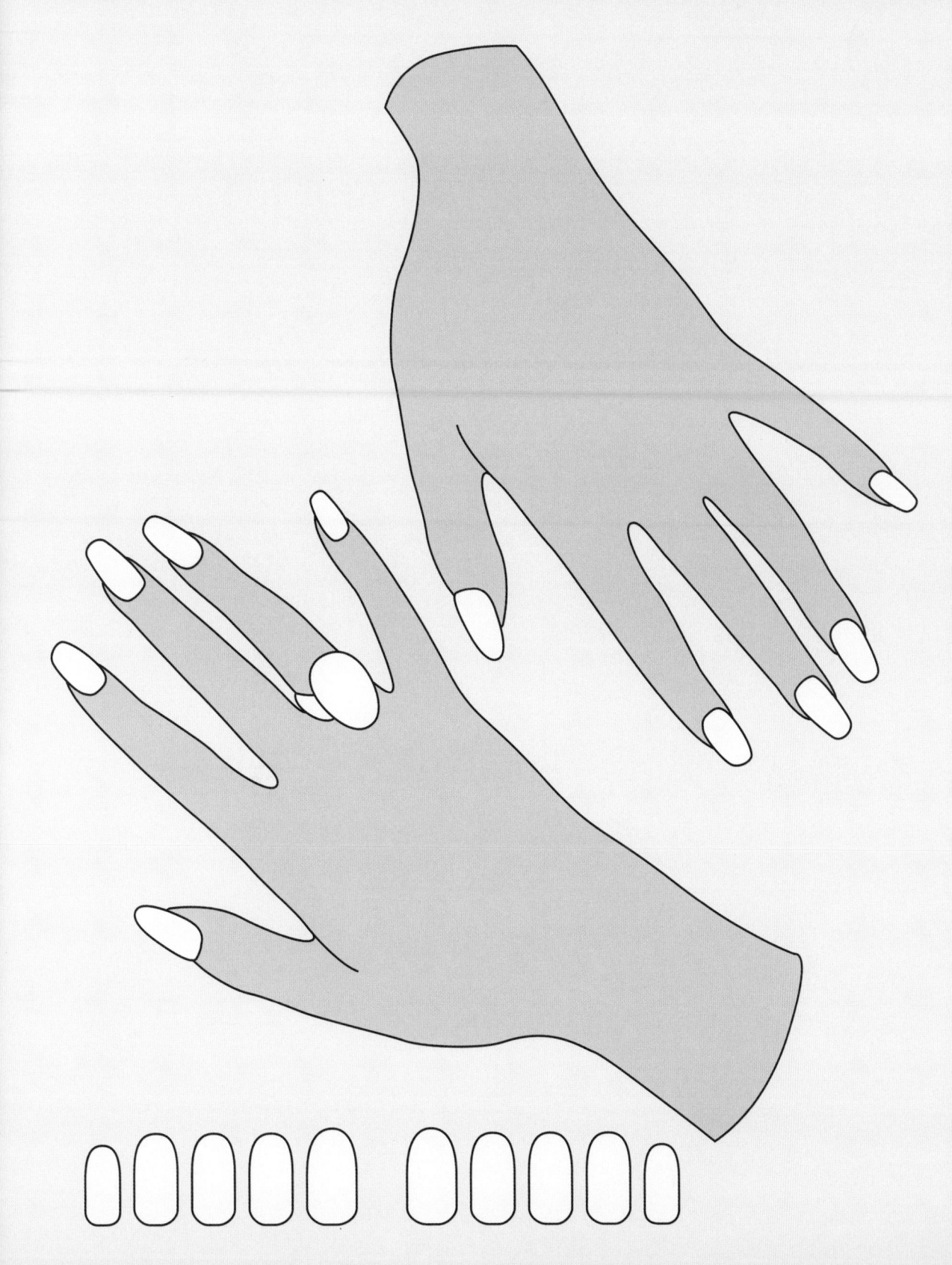

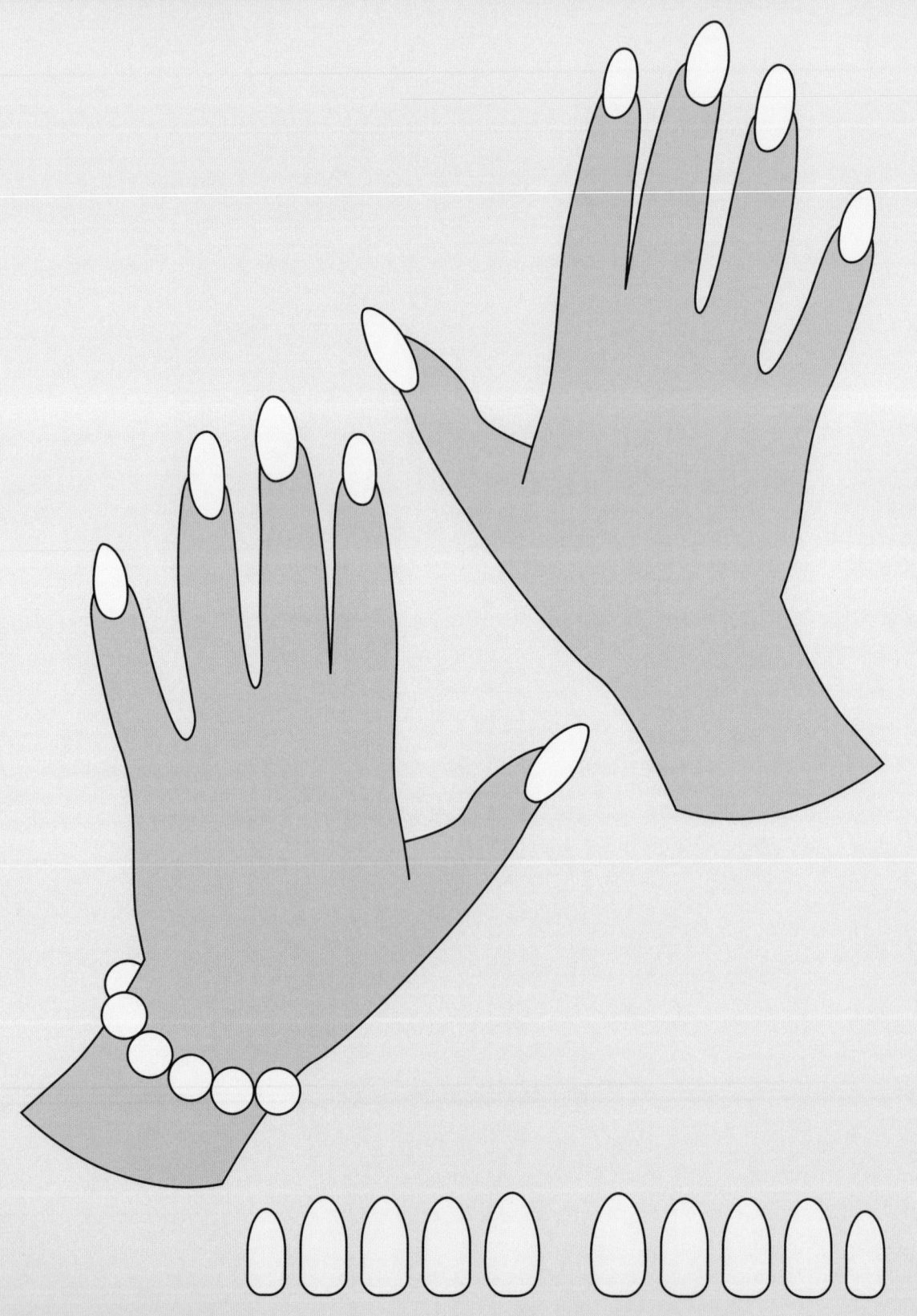

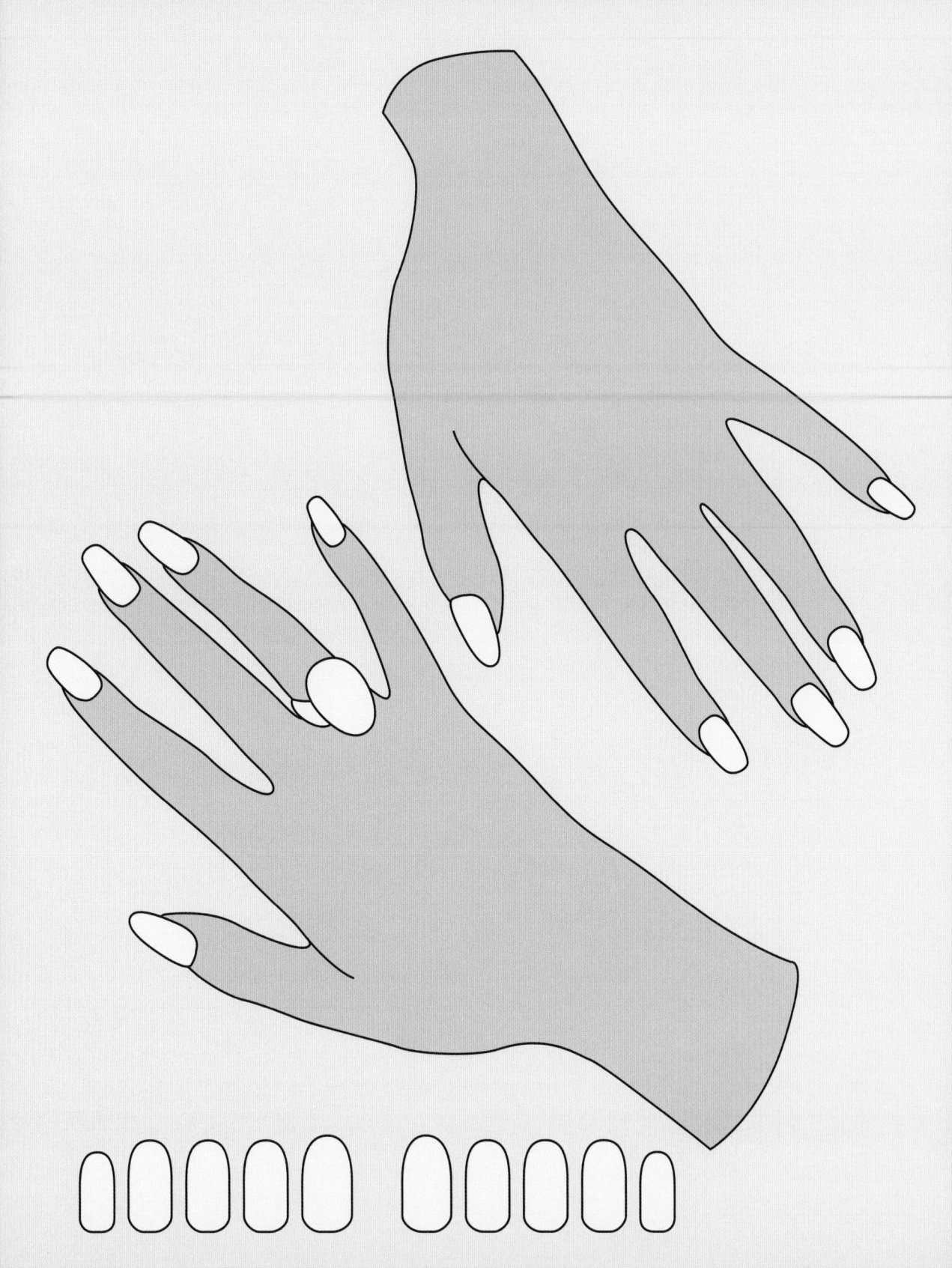

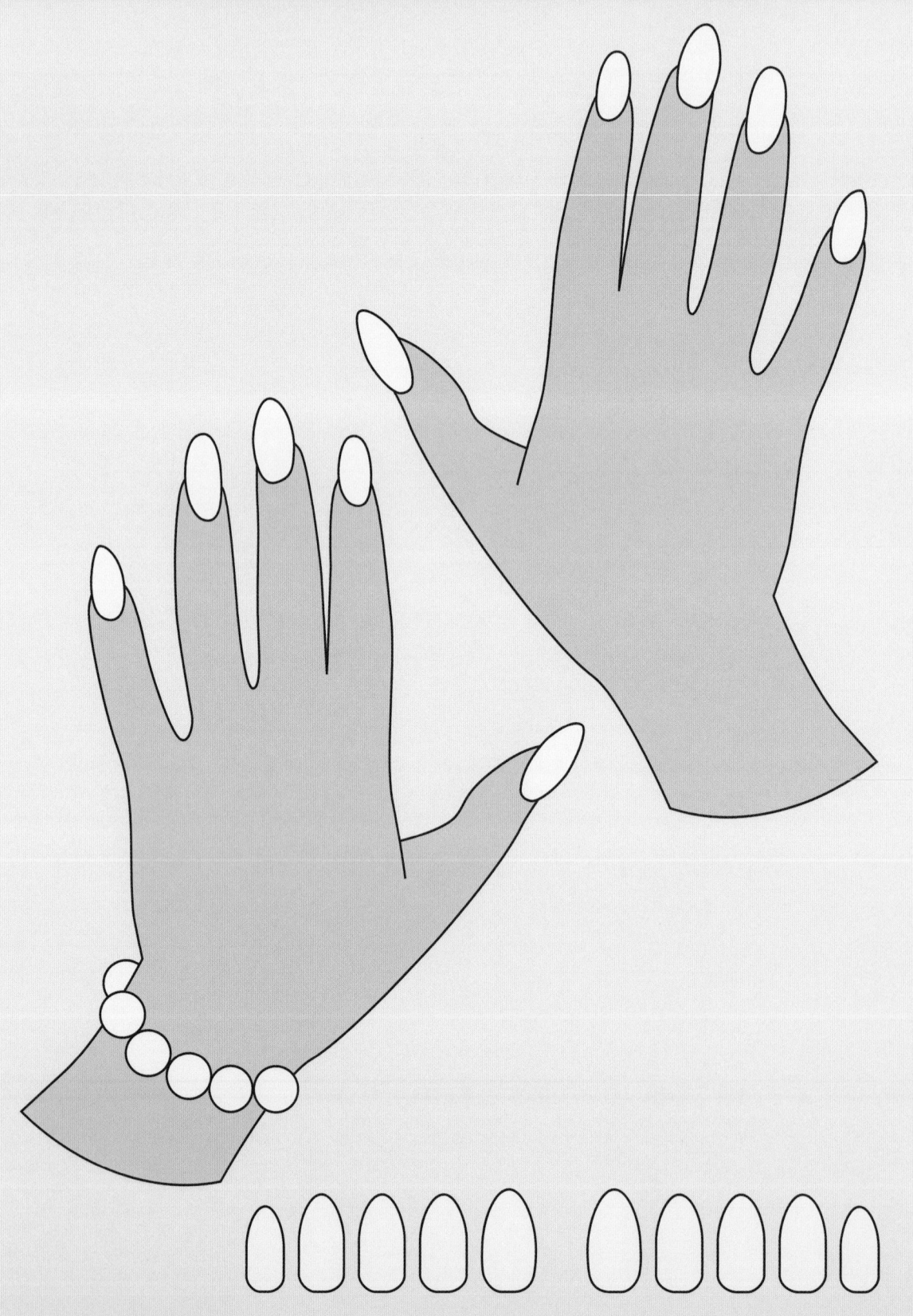

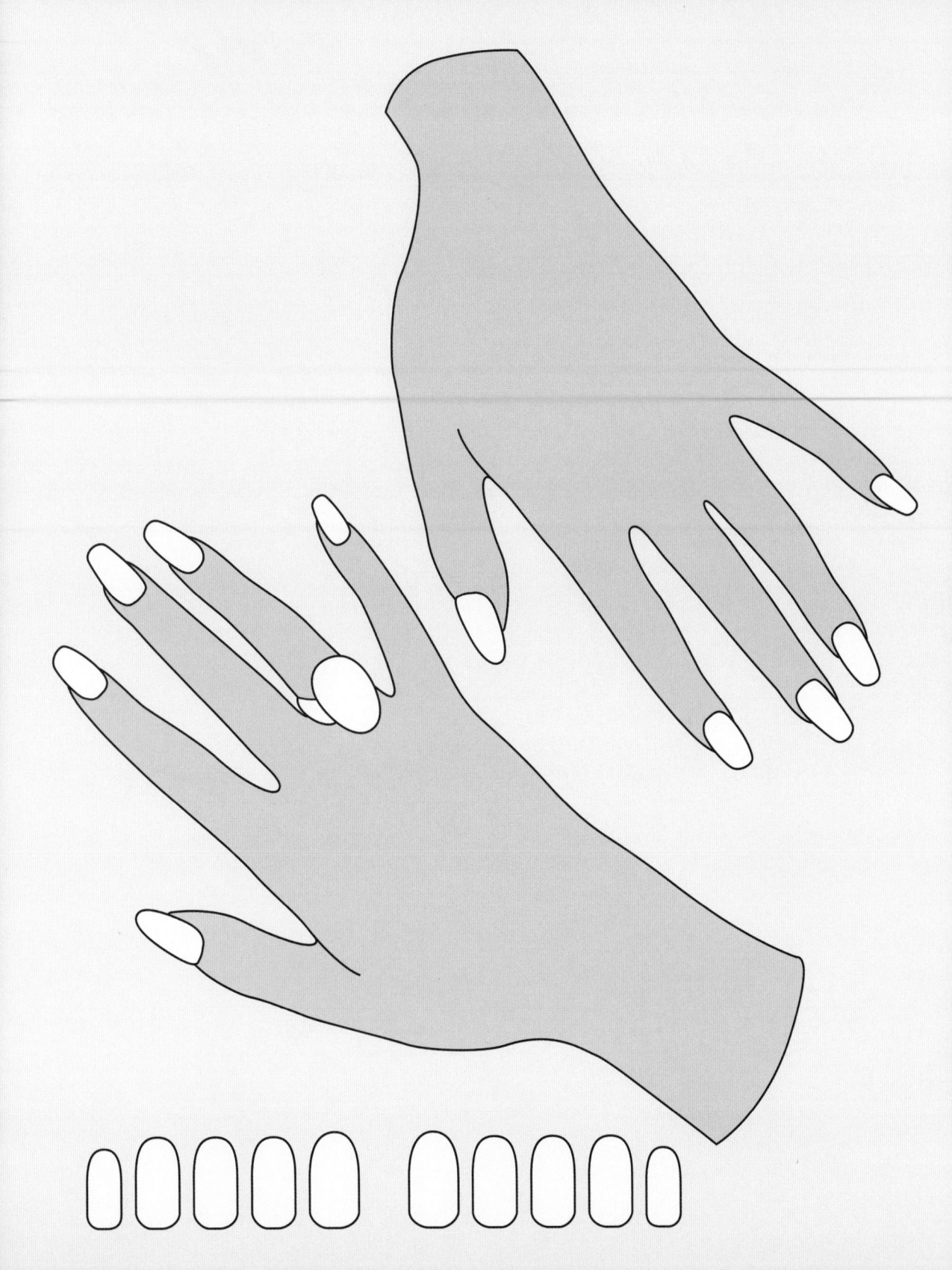

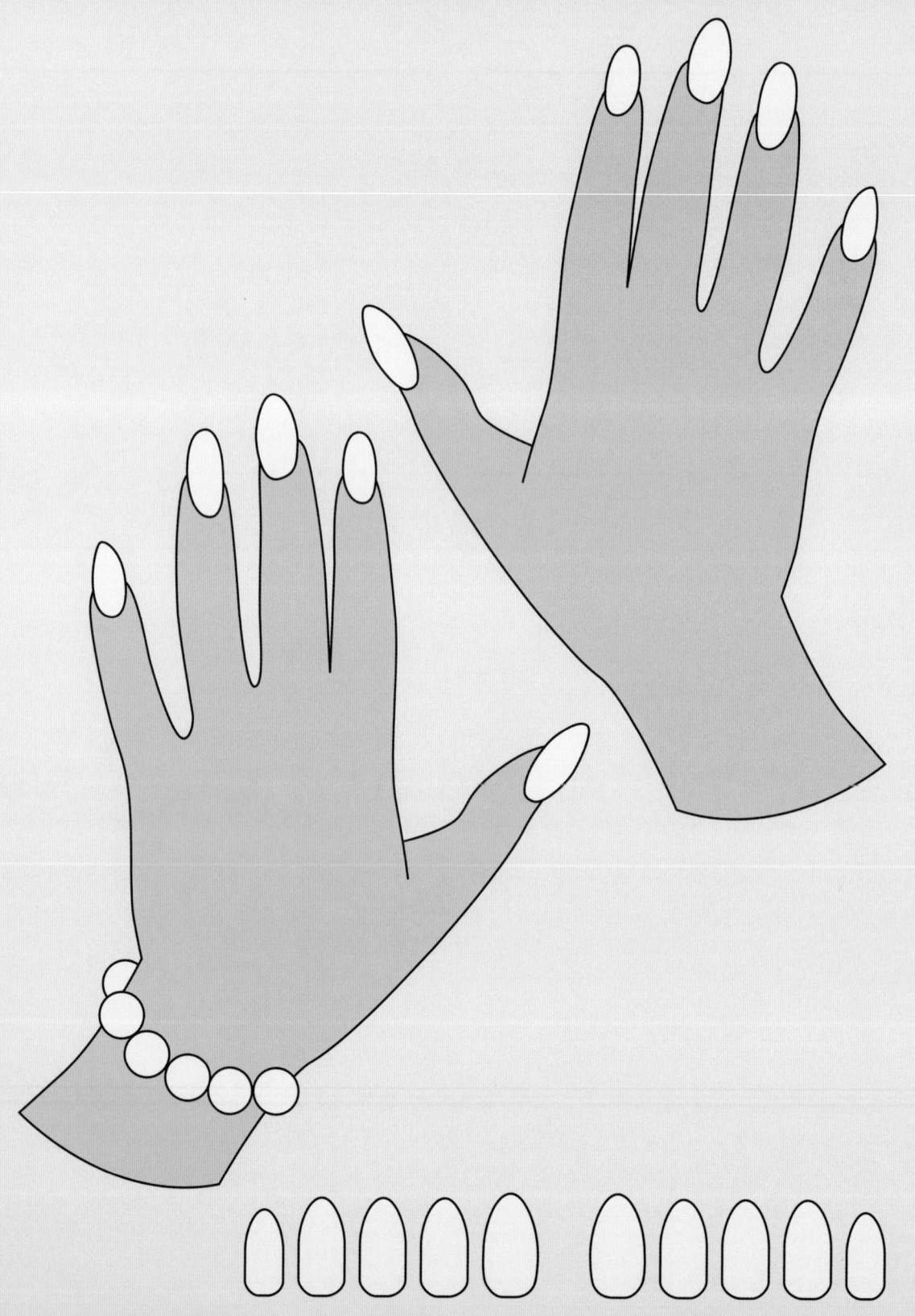

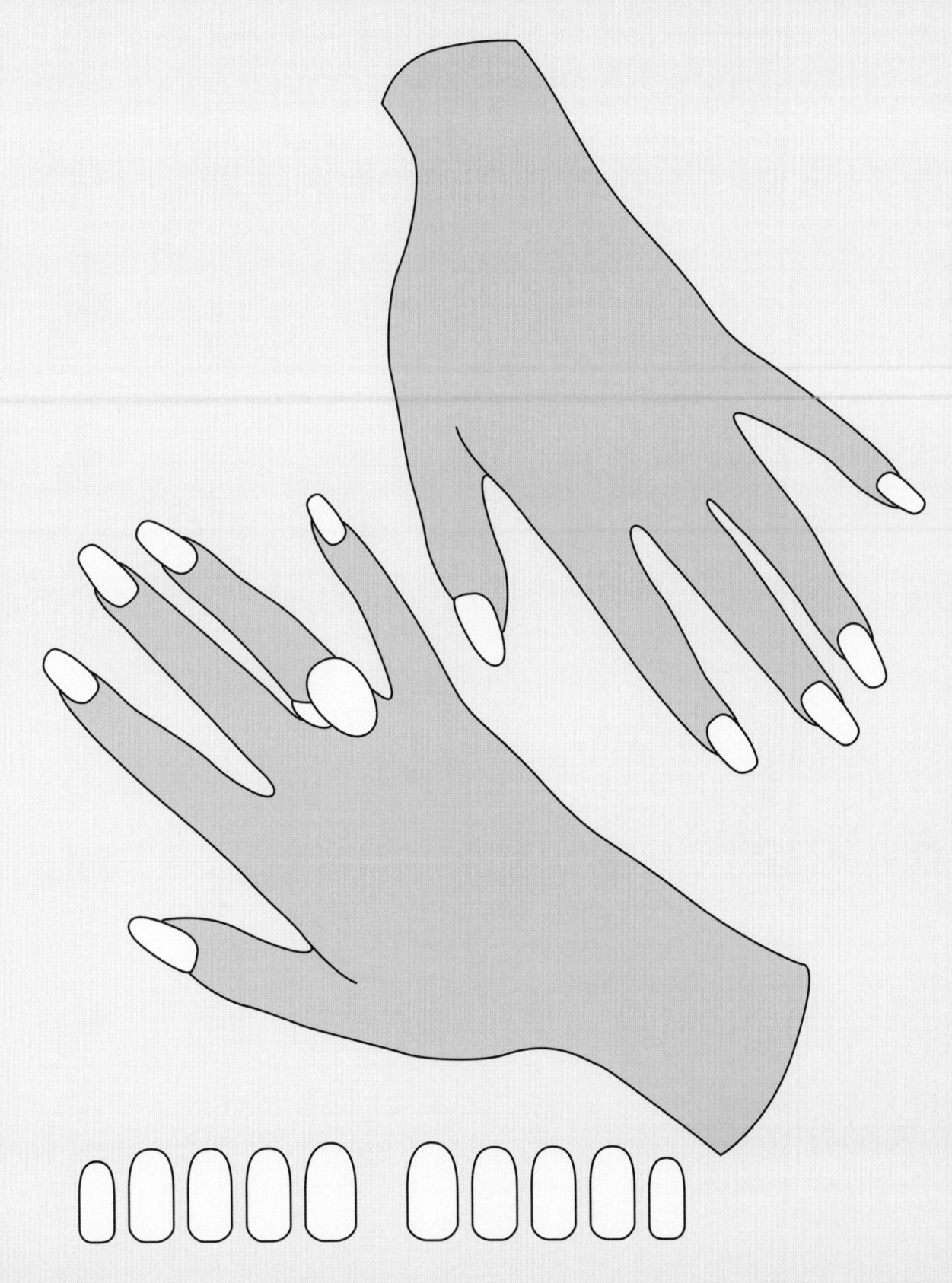

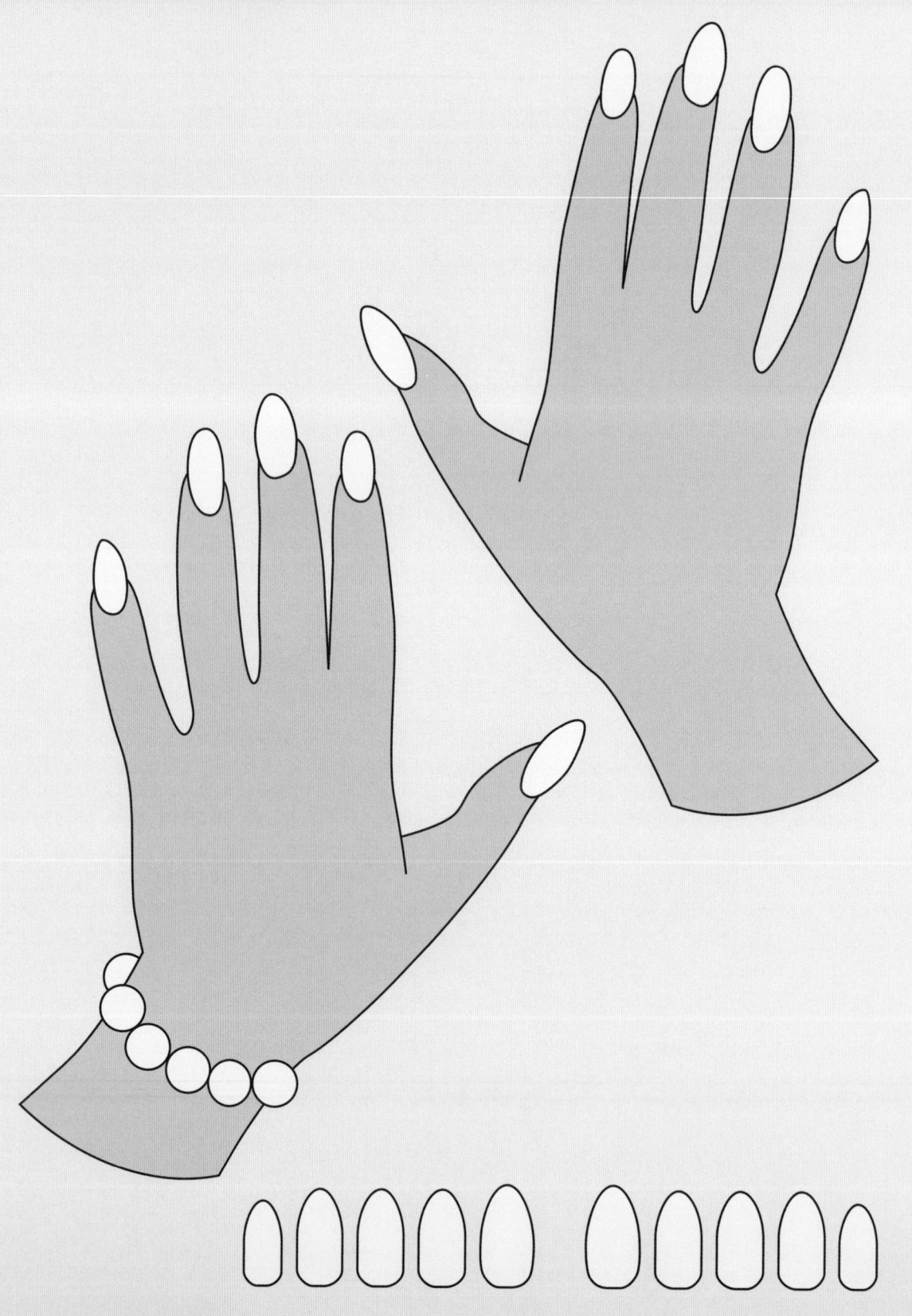

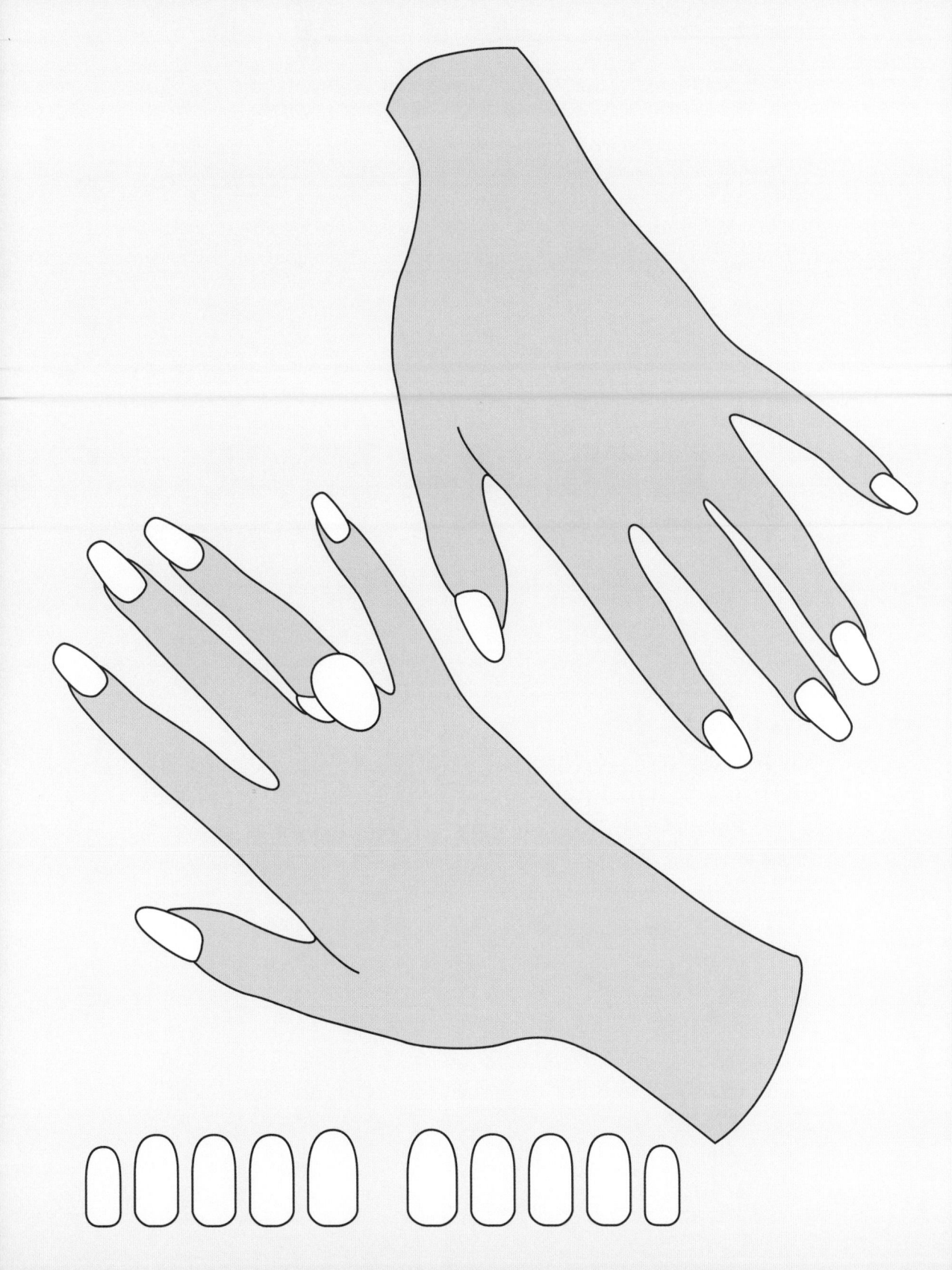

ABOUT THE AUTHOR

When I was young my mama and my aunty would sit at the corner of the dining room table while Liz, their mobile nail technician, would lay down acrylic and hand file their nails into perfectly square tips, a standard 90's nail session. She would buff away while I would reorganise her nail polish colours in rainbow order. At five years old it was like winning the lottery when, at the end of every session, she would gift me the slightly thickened bottle of a few colours that had run their course in her kit.

One night I was sneaking back and forth between the kitchen and my bedroom. Eventually my parents, curious at my scuttling around the house, came into my room to find me covered in a paste-like mix of flour and water. The result of me trying to emulate the application of acrylic powder and monomer, a type of magic that I had seen Liz perform earlier. With a plastic, watercolour brush from a dollar store craft section and a few chemical compounds missing, my dreams of long acrylic extensions ended in a scolding and a scene that I'm sure made my mama want to laugh and cry at the same time.

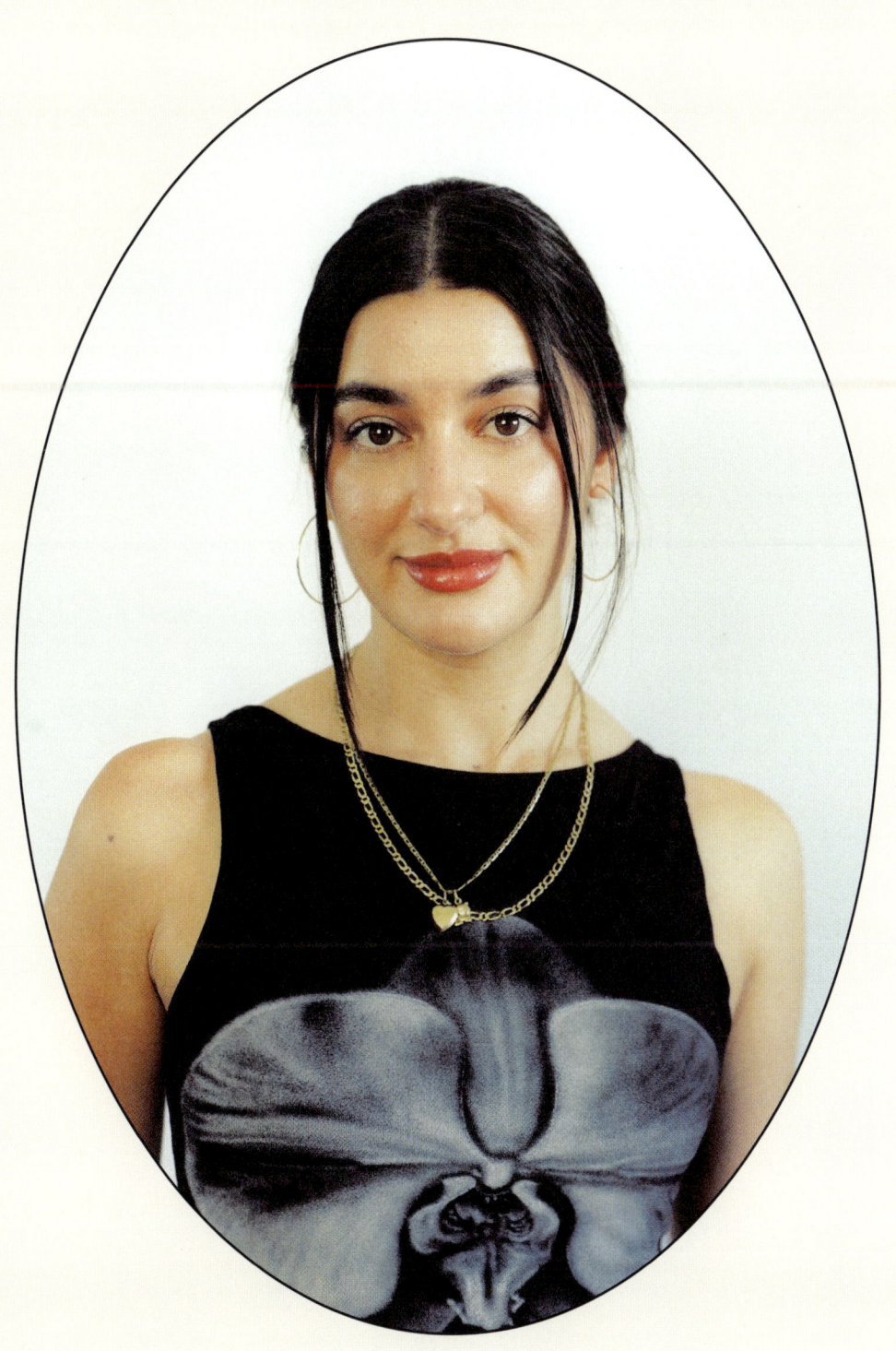

About the Author

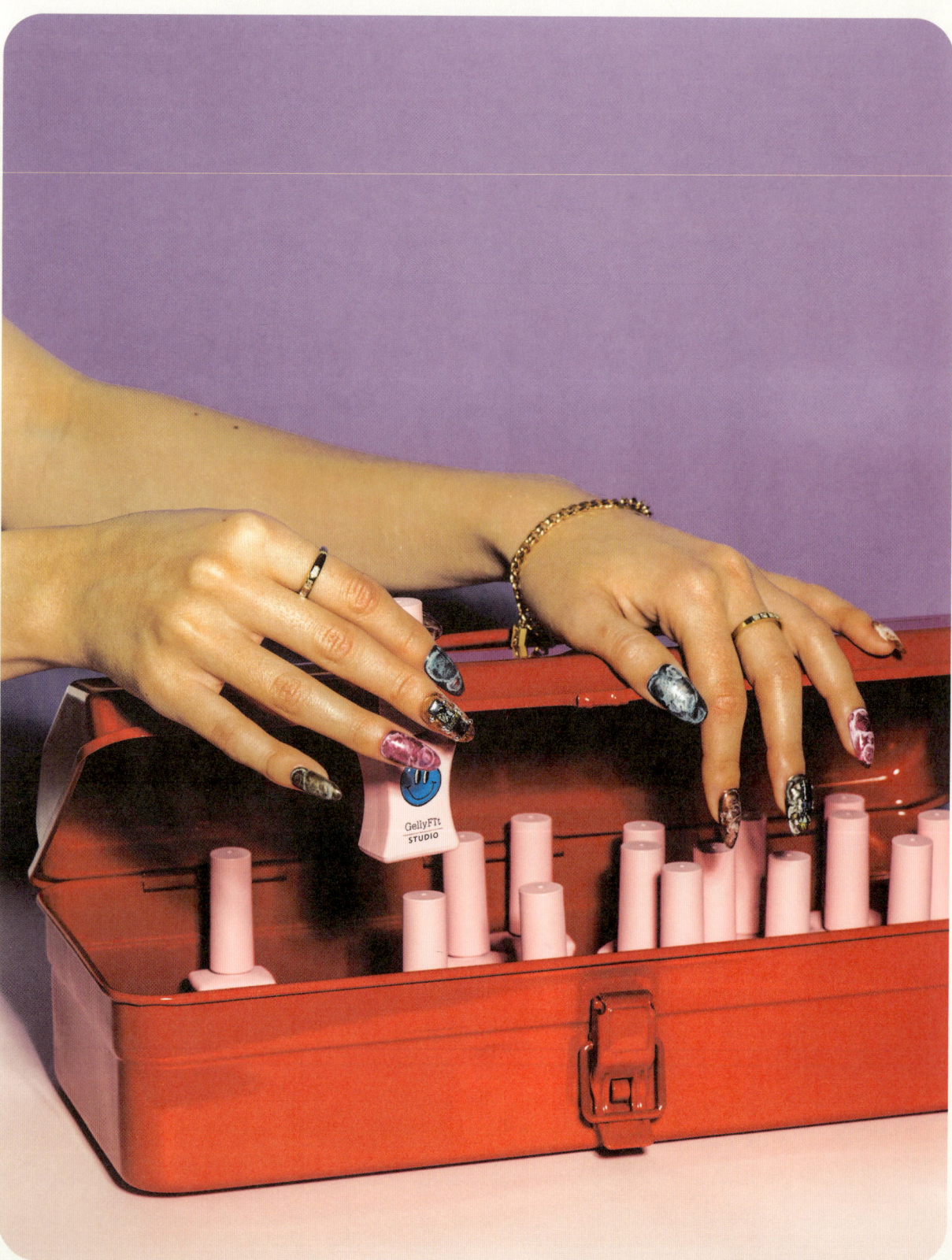

My love for nail art didn't dwindle, even when my access to the Tupperware full of flour did, even with the confines of a catholic school dress code, I found a way. If it wasn't attempting to hand paint Spongebob on one nail small enough that a teacher wouldn't spot it, it was saving up everything I had made from working Saturdays in a fast-food joint to run to a store that imported beauty goods to buy Konad stamping plates. Even when my nails were bitten nubs thanks to the stress of study, I was going to do everything in my power to make them cute again.

When I was 16, two of the most powerful forces in my life at the time met, eBay and my first debit card. They were an unstoppable pair, feeding and fuelling any and every niche hobby that spurred my interest, so it was only a matter of time before I bought my first gel, and the lamp needed to set it. Completely incapable of prepping my nails correctly, none of the sets lasted longer than a couple of days, and to this day I'm unsure of how I avoided a severe gel allergy from over exposure of all the cheapest products with the worst application. Still, the love grew, from the depths of imported nail magazines from Japan to the patience of the few friends who could bare to sit still long enough for me to attempt any kind of design on them. (This book is dedicated to you lot too.)

At 19 I worked in a shoe store and one of our sweet regulars was a woman who owned a nail salon upstairs. She offered us discounts to get our nails done and one day I booked in with a woman who kindly walked me through every step while I gawked at her precision and Japanese products and techniques, something I had only seen in a magazine up until this point. She ended up training me and within a year I had travelled to Japan and purchased my first kit.

It was years before I used the Japanese gels on anyone other than my very patient friends but that's where my aim to bring nail art to as many hands as possible began.

◉ mannequin.hands
mannequin-hands.com

ACKNOWLEDGEMENTS

With thanks to everyone who had a hand in making this book come to life.

To my dearest Georgia Softsis, nothing in my life happens without you.

To my incredibly patient and encouraging publisher, Alissa Dinallo, and the team at Sweet Hearts Press, thank you for walking me through a totally unknown experience with so much grace and generosity.

Thanks to my friends, my family and my roommates Ciarán Henry and Dulcie Tarborda for supporting me in every way, shape and form while I worked on this.

Thank you kindly to Nicole Rikos for safeguarding my sanity and calm during this process and ongoing, and to Tamlyn Edwards for keeping my body and hands in good working order.

To my dear studio mates Oscar Nimmo and Chloë Abdelnour, thank you for creating an environment so joyful, open and trusting that it could only breed creativity.

Thanks to Alana Dimou, Nyauluak Leth, Kumi Chantrill, Hannah McGrath and Mikka Byarugaba for lending their hands, skills, patience and enthusiasm to two of the most fast-paced and somehow enjoyable shoot days I've ever experienced. The imagery born of their work is at the heart of the book and without them it would have been impossible to create.

To Kurt Johnson and Steven Lattuca of Downgrade, Laura Miers, Baked in Space and Rowi Singh, thank you for lending your work and collections to the styling of the shoots: without the finer details and your beautiful work, they'd be incomplete.

Thank you, Danielle Ghazi and Jason Lung, for tediously crafting the beautiful basketball hoop that completes the studio and some of the images in this book.

And finally, with thanks to Shae Lowe for lending your skills behind the lens to this book and capturing me in a way only a best friend could.

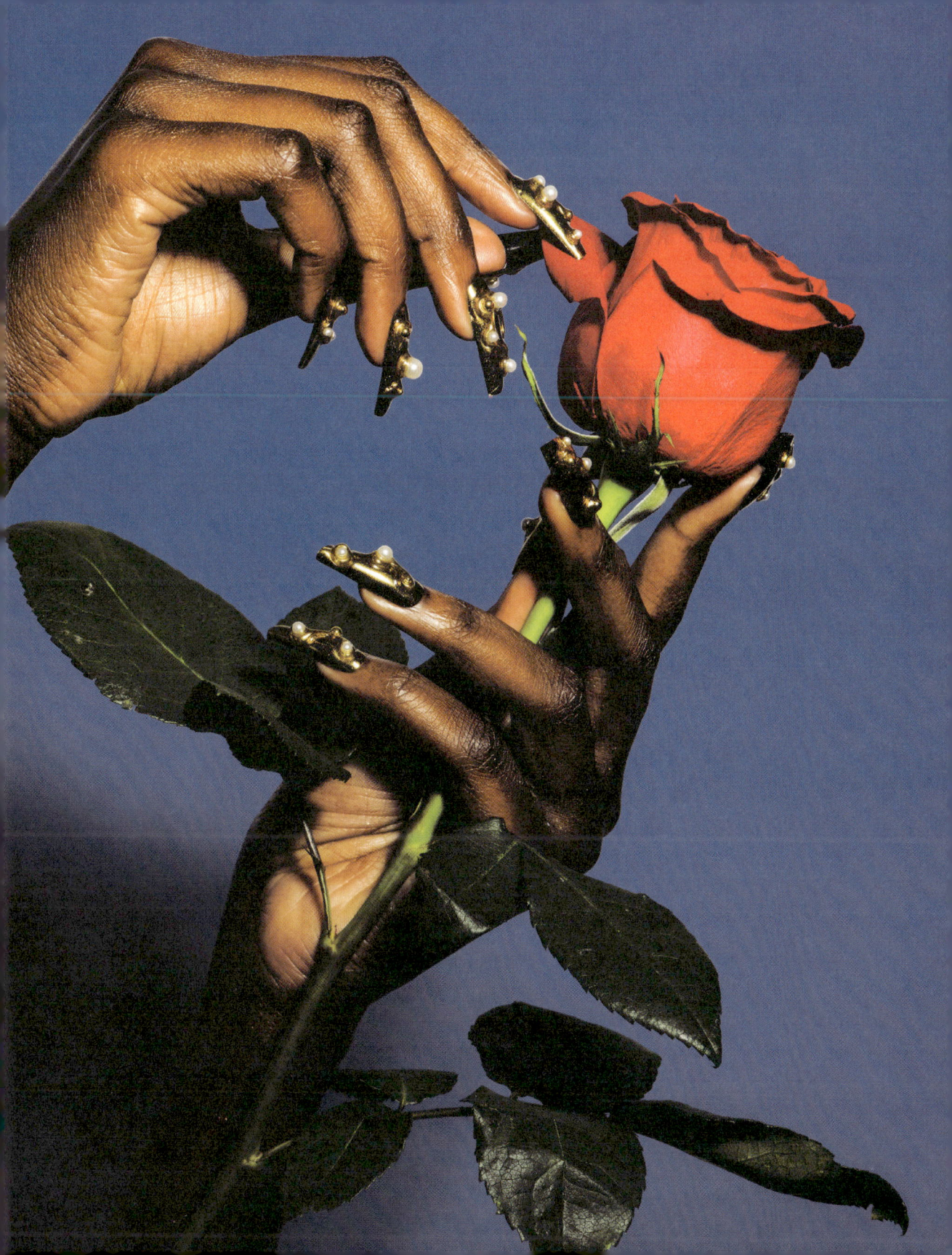

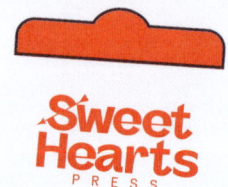

A Sweet Hearts Press book
An imprint of Rockpool Publishing
PO Box 252, Summer Hill
NSW 2130 Australia

SWEETHEARTSPRESS.COM

ISBN: 9781923208247

Published in 2025 by Sweet Hearts Press
Copyright text © Victoria Houllis 2025
Copyright design © Sweet Hearts Press 2025
Copyright chapter opener illustrations © Izzy Lawrence
Copyright photography © Alana Dimou 2025, except pages 112, 113, 120–125, 193.

All rights reserved. No part of this publication may be reproduced, stored in a retrieval system, or transmitted in any form or by any means, electronic, mechanical, photocopying, recording or otherwise, without the prior written permission of the publisher.

Text design and typesetting by Susan Le and Alissa Dinallo, Sweet Hearts Press
Cover design by Alissa Dinallo
Spot illustrations by Susan Le, Sweet Hearts Press
Photography on pages 112, 113, 120–125, 193 by Shae Lowe
Edited by Kaitlyn Smith

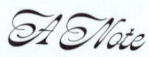

All tools should be used with care. Professional-only items should be left to the professionals and, if under the age of 18, make sure to enlist the help of an adult.

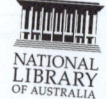

A catalogue record for this book is available from the National Library of Australia

Printed and bound in China
10 9 8 7 6 5 4 3 2 1

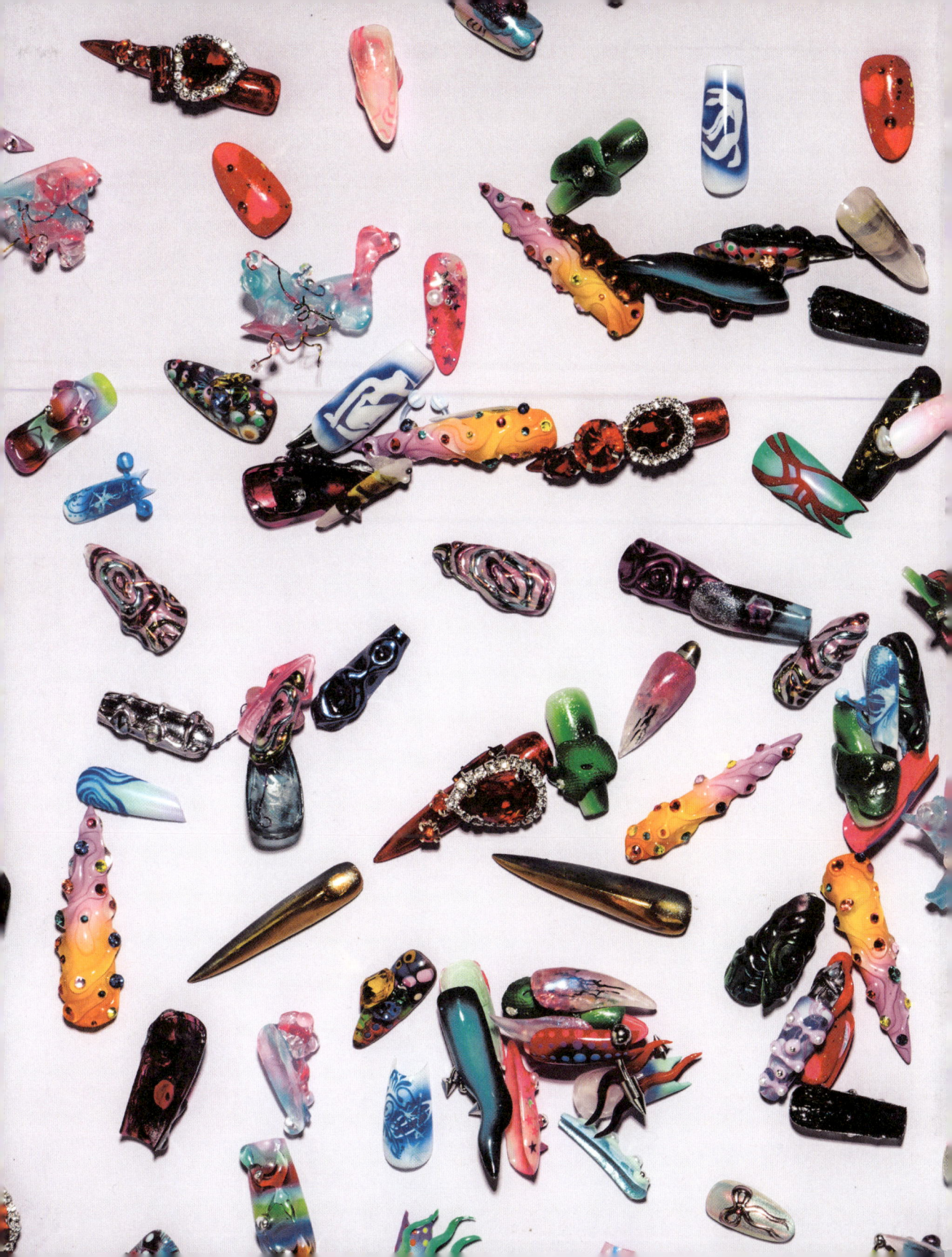

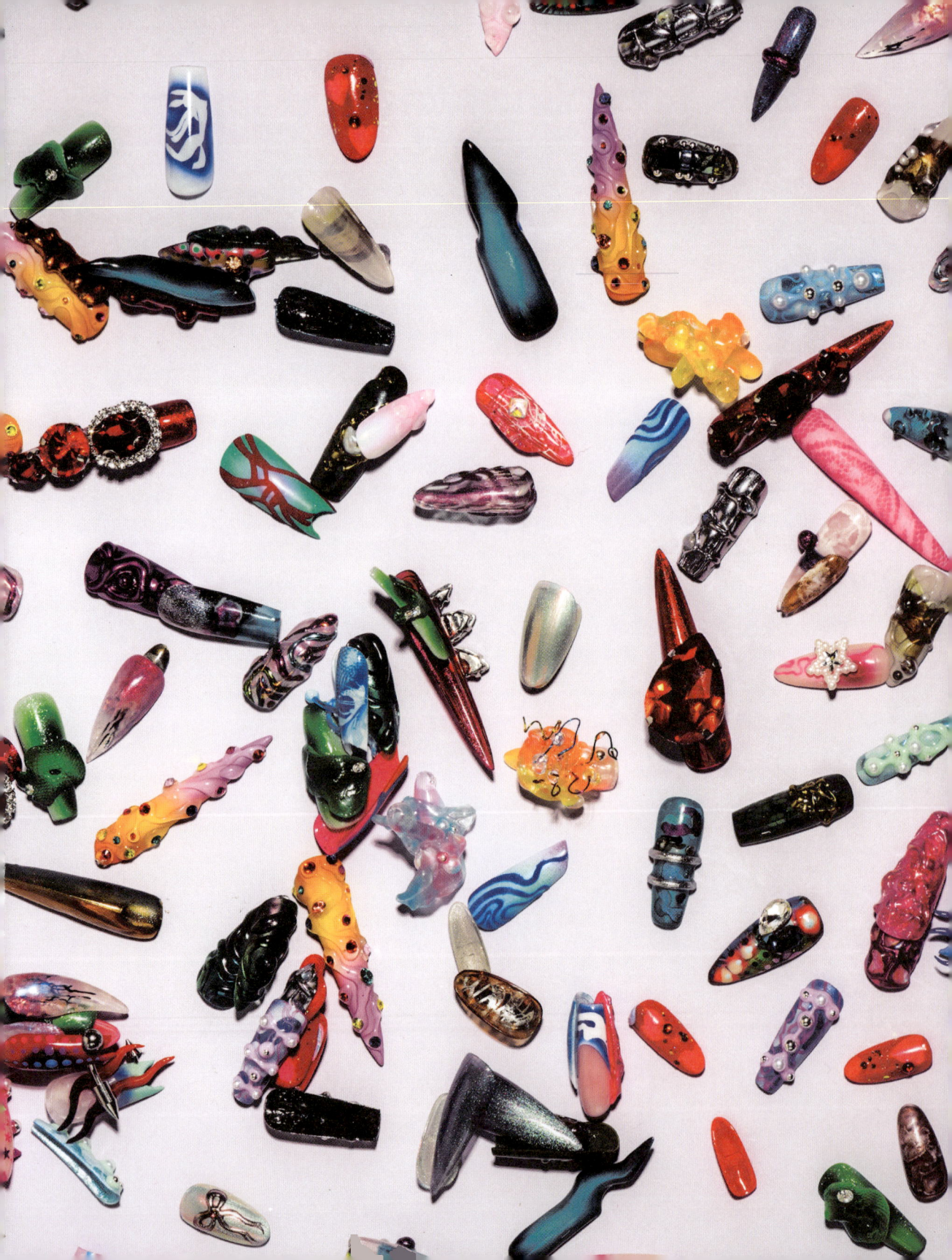